Kelly's Secrets, Rx for Longevity

"The Missing Notes"

by

John William Kelly

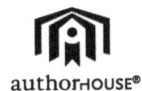

authorHOUSE®

AuthorHouse™
1663 Liberty Drive, Suite 200
Bloomington, IN 47403
www.authorhouse.com
Phone: 1-800-839-8640

First published by AuthorHouse 9/19/2007

ISBN: 978-1-4343-2481-8 (sc)
ISBN: 978-1-4343-2480-1 (hc)

Printed in the United States of America
Bloomington, Indiana

This book is printed on acid-free paper.

Contents

Chapter One: "The Missing Notes" 1

In the beginning, all the research that our pharmacist has accumulated turns up missing and something extraordinary happens.

Chapter Two: "Discovery-Time Backward" 13

In this chapter, we return to the mystery disappearance and the discovery of a youth formula that may really work.

Chapter Three: Secret #One-Safeguard The Heart 39

If the heart doesn't work, then what's the point? This chapter details how to protect and strengthen the heart.

Chapter Four: Eating Review-Kelly's Secret #Two 53

This powerful chapter is Kelly's second secret theme which covers in depth a review of foods you eat and how the processes work. In addition, the "7" factors of food are reviewed:
1-calories
2-proteins
3-fats
4-cholesterol
5-carbohydrates
6-fiber
7-sodium (salt, sod)

Chapter Five: Secret # Three-Counter Chart 71

The counter chart is a detailed list of food factors and how much of each is contained in many popular foods and meals. The lists include calories, proteins, fats, cholesterol, fiber, carbohydrates, and sodium (salt, sod)

Chapter Six: Secret # Four-Review of Antioxidants 98

This chapter includes a comprehensive review of what antioxidants do, and why they are so very important in life, health and longevity. There may be several hundred antioxidants known so far, most of which are categorized and what each one does, or is supposed to do, is discussed.

Chapter Seven: Secret #Five-Exercise Review   **125**

This chapter is perhaps the most important chapter in longevity. "The best way to reduce aging and perhaps reverse it, is to exercise". Exercise is presented in a way that gives a workable insight on how to approach exercise in a positive, easy manner.

Chapter Eight: Secret #Six-"DMVS" Dietary Minerals, Vitamins and Supplements   **135**

Taking "DMVS" (dietary minerals, vitamins and supplements) can achieve powerful abilities to reduce aging, reduce disease and prolong life. All vitamins, most dietary minerals and popular supplements are discussed, especially what they are used for.

Chapter Nine: Secret #Seven-Special Reports and Reviews Including Some of Kelly's Favorites   **169**

This chapter covers some of the most interesting articles, reviews, and research studies involving prolonged life and how to achieve it. Except for "Kelly's Favorites, One Liners", most of the reports and reviews are from various science, nutrition, medic

Why read this book: Rx For Longevity-Kelly's Secrets, "The Missing Notes"

The hope of living longer and healthier is something everyone should want, but if there's a way to reverse aging, many of us would seek it out. This book, although fiction, is based on real science and research that is available today. The hint of actually discovering a real youth formula is staggering and may lie in the secret hopes of many of us.

On the other hand, Kelly's secret notes follow a systematic approach to better health, longer life, how to lose weight, how to reduce blood pressure, how to reduce cholesterol, how to improve your heart's health, how to feel better, improve brain health, how to decrease the risk of disease, how to increase self confidence, how to look better, reduce the risk of cancer, diabetes and stroke, how to reduce muscle and joint pain, improve memory, how to make better decisions about health, and how to build up strength and increase energy.

About the author: John William Kelly, RPH

John Kelly was born in San Francisco, California. He received his B.S.(Bachelor of science) degree in pharmacy from the University of Texas, in Austin. After working 6 months as a retail pharmacist with a national drug chain, in El Paso, Texas, he attended the University of Florida graduate school for about a year, specializing in clinical pharmacology.

However, after a year of grad school, he decided to leave the academic environment and pursue a career with the drug chain. He began his career as a chief pharmacist for about a year, then he became a store manager. During his management career, he worked in 5 states and later became a district manager in Florida for nearly 20 years. During his career, he maintained several state pharmacy licenses and maintained his certifications and continuing education requirements.

All through, his working career, he would still find time to do research and at the time of his retirement, he had accumulated a massive file on health and aging. His file included encyclopedic detail on medicines from natural sources (Pharmacognosy), vitamins, antioxidants, dietary minerals and supplements. The last 2 years, while he was still working and a year after his retirement, he decided to write a book about longevity and how to achieve it.

He researched the net, especially Wikipedia, Yahoo, Google, Discover and National Geographic publications, Mayo Clinic research, various science newsletters, several nutritional publications (especially "The Complete Food Counter" by Annette Natow, PHD, and Jo-Ann Heslin, MA., R.D.), as well as publications from AARP, Wall Street Jr., Financial Times, local newspapers, USA Today and always focusing on the latest and best information about health and longevity.

This book attempts to give you solid choices and a several secrets to live longer and add some entertainment regarding the discovery of a mysterious formula that may actually reverse aging

Chapter One: "The Missing Notes"

It all began back in the 60's when Jim Kelly received a letter of congratulations and acceptance to the University of Texas at Austin, Texas. He was 16 and planning to attend pharmacy school. He was in the top 25% of his graduating high school class.

During his first early years at college, Jim wasn't any more than an average student with barely a 'c' average. There were so many exciting activities to join, it was unbelievable. He joined the glee club, karate club, university track team (he threw the javelin) and each semester, he would pick a wild elective to fill in his full schedule.

During the early years, he took Zin Buddhism, swimming, philosophy, tennis, hi-diving and even took a semester of harp playing.

It wasn't until the last semester of his second year that Jim suddenly became interested in studying seriously. Something happened. His grades the first year and first half of his second year were just passing. But beginning his second half of the second year, there was one course called microbiology. It was a huge class, with over 450 students. Jim was planning to join a professional pharmacy fraternity not just for social fun, but also, because he had heard that they kept files of all university past exams, including pharmacy exams. So by studying the previous semester exams, he should have a better chance to better perform on the current tests. Of course they were never the same. In order to join the pharmacy fraternity, you had to be passing and apply and pledge the last half of your second year.

Everyone complained about the microbiology course and how hard it was. The homework and laboratory pre-work was almost impossible. But Jim thought the course was fascinating.

The mid-term exam was just as everyone had feared, it was a disaster. The class average was 37 out of 100, with no curve. Over 450 people took the exam. As Jim walked down the hall, where the grades were posted to check his score, some of his classmates began slapping him on the his back and saying, "You son of a bitch", "Way to go", "You stinking curve buster". "Congrats, Jim", and then he saw his grade. He made an 88+, the third highest grade in the class. And the best news was, that since his lab grades were excellent, he would be exempt from taking a final.

He couldn't believe it. Wow, what a great feeling. He realized that all that studying and research not only paid off, but he felt that maybe he did have some special talent after all.

The next 3 years went well. Jim made the honor roll each semester. During his 4th year, he was assigned to take a weird course call Pharmacognosy, the study of medicines from natural sources. It was a strange course, taught by an even stranger professor of chemistry from Finland. It turned out to be one of the toughest courses in pharmacy school. But for Jim, it was another fascinating course. He loved studying "crude drugs" that were dried, unprepared natural materials used as medicine from plants and herbs. This kind of scientific research is still done today, especially in Europe and China. In fact, the Chinese were most likely the first to discover and test not only plants and herbs, but also every part of every animal and insect, searching for remedies and cures of all kinds of diseases as well as the **fountain of youth** anti-aging chemicals and miracle cure drugs.

After several days (and nights) preparing for the big mid-term, his hard work was well rewarded. Jim, not only 'aced' the exam, but he made the highest grade ever made in that course and it still stands as of today, an "A+++, an A with 3 pluses! The next day in class, the professor stopped his normal oratory and told the class he wanted to share with everyone the best test results he had ever seen in his 30+ years of teaching. He started reading the answers and to Jim's surprise, he realized it was his test. He was embarrassed, but proud. Just before the semester ended, Dr. Gjursted asked Jim if he would be interested in graduate school and working with him towards a PHD in pharmaceutical chemistry. Jim was very appreciative and said he was very interested, but after graduation, he had to work at least 6 months to pay down some of his college loans and car, and then he would decide.

Just before graduation however, Jim applied to 3 grad schools, including University of Texas at Austin, University of Michigan in Ann Arbor, and University of Florida at Gainesville. His plan was to work 6 months to a year, then attend grad school.

To his surprise, the University of Florida responded first and offered a new pilot academic program, where he could get a Masters degree in one year and a PHD degree in 2 years. At that time, the normal time was 2 years for a Masters and 3 years for a PHD. Florida also offered a monthly salary as a graduate resident plus they offered to pay all tuition and book costs. So Jim decided to go to Florida.

The first 11 months of grad school, was pure hell. In order to fit everything in, classes were a mandatory 6 days a week, Monday through Saturday and every day also had a full afternoon of laboratory class, for 11 months straight (except for a 10 day Christmas holiday). Sunday was the only day off and nothing else was possible except studying. Finally, after nearly a year, Jim decided to resign. He loved research, but the pace and academic politics was not something he enjoyed. He wanted to spend more quality time doing pure research and that just wasn't possible.

One week, before he was supposed to leave, the head of the graduate school department, Dr. Becker, called Jim over to his office. Jim had already told his immediate professors, that he was resigning at the end of the 11th month. Everyone was in disbelief. Why was he quitting? His work was very good and some of his work was outstanding. He told everyone, including Dr. Becker, that he decided that the academic world was not what he wanted to do, the rest of his life. Then Dr. Becker said, "you know Jim, I was just getting ready to place you in my PHD program, in clinical pharmacology." Everyone had high hopes for you. Your work was very good and you obviously have research talents that are excellent. Jim was stunned. He had dreamed of getting a PHD and now that it was officially offered, it was hard to believe.

Jim thanked Dr. Becker, and told him he would like to think it over that night and would check back with him the next day.
Then Dr. Becker added, Jim, I am dead serious. You have too much talent to stop now and we need you.

Obviously, Jim had a tormenting night. He tossed and turned trying to decide the best course for his career. Then he realized that he really did not enjoy teaching and that did it.
Being a college professor entails a great deal of teaching and he just didn't enjoy it.

So the next day, he thanked Dr. Becker and resumed his plans to move back to El Paso, Texas where he had worked earlier. The drug chain had repeatedly contacted him and offered him a chief pharmacist position in their best store any time he wanted.

35 years later, Jim retired! He started out as a pharmacy manager, then became a store manager and finally his last 20 years, he worked as a district manager. Although his career was management, he kept up his pharmacy licenses (Florida, Texas, Connecticut, and New Mexico), certifications and attended numerous continuing education pharmacy seminars. Back in his college days, most research was done in a lab or library. Computers were just getting started and far too expensive to use personally. But today, anyone can research almost anything, and with extreme detail. Jim's love for research never went away. He recorded many articles in his files and then went to his PDA (personal digital assistant). He loved the Palm PDA's. He faithfully transferred most of his research to his Palm and then would "sync" them to his laptop and desktop pc.

The last 2 years, while still working, Jim began to accumulate and organize his work. Then after he retired, he decided to put his research in the form of a book. During the last month, he had contacted and was corresponding with a national publisher. Jim called his wife, Mary, and said he was leaving to go and meet a publisher at the yacht club. That day would be the last day anyone would here from Jim again!

"The Missing Notes"

It was about a year later, when Mary, Jim's wife, had received a phone call about the "meeting" at the yacht club. Mary was at home, and the phone rang. A man on the phone said he would like to meet with her regarding Jim's disappearance. He went on to say that he was the publisher, at that time, and that he was supposed to meet with Jim. He said his name was Don Sutherland, and that, the day he was supposed to meet Jim, he was in a terrible car accident in Knoxville and was in the hospital for nearly a month, and when he was finally released he saw the newspaper stories about Jim's disappearance. The more he read the newspapers and television news stories, the more he thought it would be better not to get involved. He never actually met Jim and was introduced to him via an email he received from a friend of Don's, Frank Otto. Frank and Don Sutherland used to be reporters, years ago, in New York.

Mary was very reluctant at first, but decided to meet him at the yacht club in the afternoon for coffee or tea at 2 in the afternoon. Mary and Don met at the club (always lots of people there). Don was probably in his late 50's or early 60's and said he had retired from the publishing company and was now a private investigative attorney. He worked at Cooper and Cooper, one of the largest law firms in Tennessee, out of Knoxville. He went on to say, that he went to Cornell University Law School and worked as a reporter in

New York, then he got involved with a large publishing firm. Years later, he retired and moved to Knoxville and was offered a job as an investigative attorney, which he took.

Don said that when Jim talked to him on the phone (he was still a publisher then), he became fascinated by Jim's research and thought his book idea was a good one.

Don then asked Mary if anything has turned up. Mary said the police and FBI and news people were relentless for the first 6 months. There were several leads, but none worked out. Don asked her if she would like some more tea and if it would be ok to record their conversations. He said he was hired to help find any information regarding Jim's disappearance. She said ok. As they talked, Don told her that an anonymous person hired his law firm to investigate Jim's disappearance. He didn't know why. But the managing partner told him that the person who hired the firm apparently either went to school with your husband or was a co-worker at the company he worked for. He refused to give his name and insisted on remaining anonymous.

Mary then told Don that the last 2 years before he disappeared, Jim amassed a huge amount of research information and had finally contacted a publisher, you, Don.
He talked about your discussions via the telephone and internet email and that she remembered how anxious you were to publish his book because it sounded like a natural and interesting coming from a pharmacist. Don said, absolutely. What did Jim do with all his research? He kept everything written in his big black leather briefcase and copies in his Palm and his Dell laptop. When he left to meet you, he took everything with him.

Did he keep any other notes, copies or did he hot-sync the palm or laptop anywhere else? Then Mary remembered his other Palm Treo cell phone. You know, I had forgotten about his Treo phone. He always had the phone with him. He loved that phone. Mary, do us a favor and search for his phone. It's unbelievable how much information you can store in those.

What about Jim's car? It was never found and that's another mystery. How can a car just vanish? What about the internet, did he have just one email address or did he have his own website? I don't think so. We shared the laptop everyday and he would always teach me or show me anything new. The FBI searched everything. We only have one email address, as far as I know.

Mary, you seem to be handling everything alright. It must have been really tough. Yes, I was a mess for at least 6 months. My son and relatives all came down and stayed with me as much as they could until I somewhat recovered. Then I decided to go back to work part time and that helped the most. I am also a pharmacist, a hospital pharmacist. So I work ½ days, 3 days a week.

Mary, do you have a desktop computer? Maybe Jim hot-sync'd his research on that computer. I don't think he did, but you are welcome to check. The desktop is several years older, but he did upgrade it Microsoft XP. You know Don, now that we talk about this, I remember Jim saying, about 2 weeks before he disappeared, that he believed he discovered something.

What do you mean Mary? Well, he said something was "working". One of his discovered secrets was working. Please continue Mary. Well, Jim used to dye his hair and moustache every 3 weeks. He said his hair and moustache, after 6 weeks didn't need to be dyed. His dentist said his gums and teeth appeared remarkably improved and healthier. Also, he just looked a little better. That sure sounds interesting. I remember now, when he talked on the phone, that he sounded excited and even a little nervous.

Mary, can you recall if Jim discussed his work with anyone else? Maybe he talked to a relative, golf buddy, or friend. Well there was this one guy who called him about 3 weeks before he disappeared and they were on the phone for hours. I thought it may have been you, the publisher, but Jim said it was someone he thought he knew at first, but it wasn't him and the caller sounded foreign, probably from Asia or the Middle East.

The caller kept asking Jim so many questions and then asked him if he needed any financial backing or money to help with any of his research. Jim was surprised the person knew about his book. How could he know anything about his research or the book? Who told him? Even Don, the publisher, only had a non-detailed overall picture of what the book was about. Don then said, yes that was true and we thought the concept of a publishing a pharmacist's knowledge of health and longevity would be a winning combination for readers. Everyone trusts their pharmacists!

Mary, do you remember anything else? Mary replied, no, not at the moment. Let's go back to the desktop computer. Do you know how to look up file names? Mary said no. One easy way, is to check your icons and see if a folder with a name is present. If not, click on start, click on all programs, check under documents and Microsoft word, then click on file, open see the list of documents. Look for the file names. Don, that's not my thing. Let's do this. My son, Mike, will be in tomorrow, all day. Why don't you come over and meet him and you both can check out the desktop pc. He is a whiz with computers.

Mary, here's my business card with my cell numbers and office number. Please call me any time, night or day if I can help or if you find something. Now Mary, before we conclude today, do you remember anything else? Mary replied, not at this moment, but do you think this person that hired your law firm is the same person that called Jim? Don said, good question, and believe me we will find out and I'll personally discuss it with you.

Mary, I am sorry, but I do have a few more questions. Who was the FBI agent in charge and lead police officer who worked with you? Marlin Becker was the special agent in charge and here's his number. The main police lieutenant in charge was Chris White and here is his number. Is it ok with you if I contact these officers? Mary said yes, of course.

What about your son, Mike? What did he have to say about all this and where was he when Jim disappeared? My son was in Suzhou, China teaching English and just returned for 3 weeks during the investigation, then he went back to China to finish out the year and came back last month to enter graduate school at the University Of Tennessee. Mary, would it be ok to talk to him? Mary said yes, and you can talk to him tomorrow.

Don, what do you think happened? Gosh Mary, I don't know. It's the most bizarre case I have ever heard of. It's like he just vanished. Mary, there's lots of water around these lake roads, has anyone checked to see if he could have driven off the road into the lake? Mary said, yes, they had boats with divers and detectors testing the entire area and the highway department along with the police checked all the nearby roads for skid marks, and damage. Nothing was ever found.

What about the yacht club? Did they have any reservations for Jim and I? We were supposed to meet at 2 pm. Yes Don, Jim made the reservation, but no one came. So, something happened to both of us on the way to the club. Wow, what a mess. Mary, I am really sorry about this. I want you to know, we will do everything possible to find Jim and what happened to him. Wait a minute, Mary said! I just remembered Jim's "code". What code, what do you mean? Well, when Jim was district manager, he would test all his employees to see if they knew the cost of the merchandise. I believe they used a pricing code called "Brushclean", which was a letter code equal to the numbers, 1 through 9 and the last letter, n was 0. Jim rarely trusted anyone, except me, and he would do all of his passwords in Brushclean code. Say you wanted to use a password of 911. Then I believe the code would be abb. That's the example Jim would always use, so that I could easily remember. And I seem to recall that he said he was going to send his research via Microsoft Word in a folder called "Seven L's" which referenced his seven secrets. Let's see, that would be "LLLLLLL" in Brushclean code. Tomorrow, when you and Mike check out the desktop computer, hopefully you can discover something.

The next day, Don met Mike and then quickly asked Mary and Mike if he could talk to them outside the house. Don suggested that when they go back inside the house, that they should not talk outloud. The house could be bugged. Remember, Mary, your husband didn't just disappear. Also, remember that I am your attorney and that anything we find is confidential. Do we all agree? They agreed. As Mary looked on, Mike and Don went through all the computer "folders" looking for clues. They couldn't believe how many there were. Finally, hours and hours later, and when they were just about to give up, they discovered a folder called "Kelly 7". Mike, a computer geek, said it looked like what we were looking for. Sure enough, after he tried to open it, using the password, LLLLLLL, and it worked. Open sesame! Wow, it was hard to contain there excitement and they all reminded each other to be quiet and not talk. There it was. The file opened and there was Jim's "Missing Notes", nearly 200 pages of glorious research. It was all typed and ready to send and or copy. Mike said it would be safer to copy on data discs and also, send or email to each of us as a backup.

The decision was made by Mary, to have emails sent to Mary, Mike and Don as an attachment requiring a special code to open. After that was sent, then the book would be copied on data discs. Don then pointed to the door and that they all go back outside to discuss. First, the discovery was to be kept absolutely secret between the 3 of them only. Don, being a veteran attorney, suggested they make it official and he would ensure that no one, including his firm, would find out about the 'book'. Don also recommended that Mary should be in charge of whatever decisions are made regarding any further actions. Don reminded them, that it remains critical that everyone stay confidential. Something happened to Jim. He just didn't vanish. There may be some person or persons or agency involved that may still be watching your activities. If you do notice anything out of the ordinary, call me on my cell night or day, even the smallest change.

A week later, Don met with Mary at the yacht club for lunch and discussion. Mike was invited, but he had an exam and had to work after that. Don said, no problem, that he would catch up with him later and bring him up to date, if that's ok with Mary.
Mary said ok.

As Don began to go over the 'book', with Mary, he recommended that she proof read it and make any changes and she should become the 'co-author', officially. Mary was also a current licensed and certified pharmacist and her expertise would add to the 'books' credit and give the publisher a great book to release. Mary said, it's what Jim would have wanted. He really wanted to give back to the public and help others develop a healthy lifestyle, especially, but not exclusively, Americans. Mary said she would proof read it and that they should meet again the following week and Mike should also attend.

Mary was amazed how detailed and interesting the 'book' was. She knew Jim had spent hundreds, maybe thousands of hours researching, but had never taken the time to review or read his work. Some of the reports and guidelines were so down to earth and important, she decided to follow most of them immediately.

The next week, they all met and Mary stated that this book had to be published. It was too important. Don said, that if it was ok with her and Mike, he would set everything up with one of the best publishing companies. He would review the publisher's contract with them for their approval. Mike said, it's Mom's book now, she should make all the decisions. Ok, then we are all agreed?!

6 months later, the book became a national best seller. Mary consented, for awhile, at least, to attend several signings, and even some television talk shows. The popularity of the book combined with the drama of Jim's mysterious disappearance was a perfect

recipe for sensationalism. But beyond that, the sensationalism might be just the thing needed to find Jim and or what happened to him.

Chapter Two: "Discovery-Time Backward"

Six months after Mary released the 'book', it became a national best seller. Mary as 'co-author' was now traveling constantly. She already attended dozens of book signings and was scheduled to appear on more television shows. The combination of the mystery disappearance and the secret to possibly halt aging was an absolute firecracker.

Now, almost a year after publication, she began to detest all the traveling and sensationalism. But, it sure helped her banked account, which blossomed some several million dollars plus. Mike, her son, only had one more semester to go and he would finish graduate school. She was so proud of him. He has already had several offers from great companies. Mary was just hoping he wouldn't take a job too far away and leave her alone in Tennessee. But she would be supportive no matter what he chose.

Mary decided to stop all the traveling and spend more time relaxing in her new lake home and her new boat. The home she purchased came with a fantastic covered boat dock with an easy lift. Mary and her son Mike picked out a new Chapparel 26 foot inboard/outboard deck boat. She joined the local boat club which meets once a month on the second Wednesday of each month. All the boat owners and their families boat up to the Blue Heron Island campground for some serious barbecuing and socializing.

On Mary's second campground outing, she decided to go alone. Mike was in class and Don Sutherland and his wife were on vacation. The Sutherlands became close friends. Last month, Mike and Mary attended three afternoon classes of the Coast Guard Auxiliary boating course and it was so interesting. It was a fun course and it gave great tips on boating safety and how to handle boats.

It was about 10:00 in the morning when Mary pushed her boat away from her dock. She brought a picnic lunch, lots of drinking water, and before leaving, she made sure to do her Pre-launch check. Gas was near full, all the life vests (also called personal floatation devices), were out and unsealed. She also made sure she had a working flashlight, safety flares, orange signal flag, first aid kit, boat hook, portable GPS and marine radio. She carried the GPS device and the marine radio in her pocket book. The GPS shows the longitude (pole to pole) and latitude (around or equator, or lateral) positions. So, if something happens, it will show her exact location anywhere on earth.

The marine radio is also very important to broadcast an emergency message. Channel 16 is the emergency channel and when used, it will notify the Coast Guard and emergency services. By law, if you are underway, the marine radio must be turned on.

As Mary neared the starboard side (right side) of the main channel buoys, she mentally rested and couldn't believe how beautiful the lake and surrounding area was. It was so peaceful. She only had to go another mile or so to the campground or if she changed her mind and wanted to go to the yacht club and dock, it was just down the lake on the other side. As she stood and turned around to view the scenic gorgeous day, she noticed another deck boat behind her picking up speed. No problem, it was 'Boat Wednesday' and many boats would take this way to head for the campground or yacht club.

As the boat got closer, Mary couldn't help but notice the handsome young man at the helm. He was probably in his early 30's. She was 57. Oops! She shouldn't stare. As the boat neared, she couldn't take her eyes off him and she couldn't figure out why. My God!, it looks like Jim, 35 years ago! Boats are to stay at least 50-150 feet away from other boats while underway. As the young man pulled within about 50 feet, he turned to Mary and smiled and quietly waved hello. Mary, blushed, smiled, and waved back.

Then suddenly, her marine radio blared, "ahoy there, please switch to channel 68". That voice sounded like, no, it couldn't be! Then she heard, "Mary, take hold of yourself, its Jim"! Mary nearly fainted and burst into tears. Mary, Mary, snap out of it, I don't have much time, so please listen. Let's drive over to the Tanasi boat ramp and meet there. Try to act normal. Are you alright? Can you do that? Go slow and I'll follow you and let's not talk on the radio. Ok? Mary said ok.

Mary just couldn't believe her eyes and she couldn't stop shaking. He looked and sounded just like Jim looked back when they first got married, some 35 years ago. How could this happen and what has Jim done? They cruised about 20 miles per hour until they approached the dock area to tie up. They slowed to no wake speed and as they neared the docks, Jim pointed to the dock where no other boats were parked and there were no people around.

Mary threw out her 'fenders' (cushions to keep the boat from touching the ramp or dock). She carefully stepped out and tied the deck ropes to the nautical poles. Then Jim came over and docked and they embraced. It was a cautious embrace. Mary wasn't convinced it was Jim and Jim looked somewhat nervous, like someone might see them. Jim told Mary to go over to the tables with an umbrella and pick one where no people were around and they would talk.

As they sat down, Mary was still shaking and Jim tried to calm her down. Mary, I can't imagine what's going through your mind right now, but I can only stay a short while, so please listen carefully. Mary tried to pull herself together and wiped the tears away and began to listen to Jim's story.

Mary, last year, I was on my way to meet the publisher, Don Sutherland, at the yacht club. When I pulled up to park, a big black SUV pulled up close to my car and three guys got out. They were well dressed in suits, and said they wanted to speak to me. They looked like FBI types, except they were foreigners. They showed me some identification cards and badges and told me that King Mohammed Alabbar Rashid, III, is in the car and he would like to speak to me in private. Nobody seemed hostile or aggressive. I said, well what's this about? They said they didn't know what or why the King wanted to speak to me, but he wanted to meet me. He is in the car, if you would like, King Rashid will come out and talk to you. I said yes, I would be prefer that.

King Rashid was a big man, older and probably in his late 70's and except for the grey beard, he was dressed impeccably. He quietly, but firmly told his staff to go inside the club house and he would summon them after we talked. His mannerisms and voice indicated he was very cultured and well educated.

Well Mr. Kelly, it's truly a pleasure to finally meet you. Would you like to speak here or in the car? We can roll down the windows or leave a door open if you wish. Well, why don't you start off and tell me what this is all about? It's about your research! I am very interested in your 'book'! How could you know anything about my book? I haven't told anyone!
Then the King went on to say, that I may have talked to someone, like my next door neighbor, Bruce. He told me about your book.

You know your neighbors operate one of the largest security companies in the world. They have operations in over 20 countries, including mine. I recently hired them to bid on the security services on some of my oil operations. When we went out to dinner one night, we were talking about getting old and wish we could reverse it, and then Bruce told me about you and the book you were writing. He said you were writing a book about living longer, that you were a pharmacist and it was kind of weird, but he thought you were looking younger. We talked more, and he said you were a very smart person, the research, studious type. He went on to say, that you were recently retired and were probably an expert on vitamins and drugs. So, Mr. Kelly, that is why I am here.

Why don't we sit in the car? I said ok. Mr. Kelly, let me begin by saying that I have come from a long line of kings. My family has owned large interests in the Middle East for over three centuries. I have amassed a great personal fortune that would put your Mr. Bill Gates to shame. I own several financial institutions, large real estate investments, many corporate companies as well as massive oil properties. My family is very large and I have seven sons. Only one of my sons has the ability, trustworthiness and intelligence to carry on my empire. Unfortunately, last year, he and his family were killed in a suspicious boating accident. All my other sons and their families are greedy, wasteful and probably have already planned my 'accidental demise'. If there is any chance you have discovered a way to live longer, perhaps I can outlive my greedy sons and pick one of several worthy grandsons. How much money would you take for some of this youth formula?

King Rashid, I don't know. I hadn't thought about it in that way. I was hoping to make some money off the publication and release of the book. I figured if it was a success, I might be lucky enough to make a million or two.

Mr. Kelly, I will offer you a billion dollars if it works and pay the taxes, if you give me your secret. I can also set you up a laboratory, or set up any computer system you desire. My only requirement is that you come back with me to Dubai and stay with me for one month to test your formula and see if it really works. Or if you prefer, you can stay at my retreat in West Palm Beach, I have a large home and yacht there. It is very private there. In addition, if you accept my offer, you must leave at once with me and cannot talk to anyone, including your family and friends.

After one month, you may return to your home and family, but no one must ever know what happened or my name must not be involved. I must also tell you, your family may already be under surveillance. My sons are also very wealthy and can easily afford to hire any company to investigate or follow anyone. You would never know your were under surveillance.

Also, in the event your formula doesn't work on me, I will still deposit the sum of ten million dollars and tax payments in your bank account.

King Rashid, why all the secrecy? And I can't just take off and leave my family without any notice and why do I have to go with you? Mr. Kelly, think about what you are doing. If anyone finds out that you may have discovered a miracle to halt and perhaps reverse aging, what do think would happen? People would stop at nothing to get your formula. You couldn't handle the amount of money people would be willing to pay. And there are many groups of people that would do anything to stop you and kill you and your family because of some of the religious and moral implications. You wouldn't be safe staying here and your family could be kidnapped and probably killed. No, the only answer is for you to 'disappear'.

Now before you decide, I need to know as honestly as possible, does your formula work? You know, according to my information I have on you, it states that you are 63 and I can tell you, you don't look at day over 40. How old are you? I am 63.

Before I decide anything, I have to be convinced that my family will be protected. King Rashid agreed. Secondly, I will never give my formula to anyone, not even you. However, I may allow someone, like yourself, to test it, under my control. You should be able to see some results within 30-60 days. By the same token, everyone is different. The results may not be the same. It may take longer or not work at all, depending on your diet, genetic makeup and your specific lifestyle. But, after a trial period, you will know one way or another. Also, I am not interested or willing to go to any foreign country. The Palm Beach idea sounds more workable, but again, I just can't see how I can just leave my family and not tell them.

Mr. Kelly, it's for their protection! And besides, who knows how many people your neighbors told and they travel all over the world.

Also, according to what your wife told your neighbor, she said that she noticed that you were looking healthier, younger and that your grey hair had disappeared!

Look, Mr. Kelly, I will personally promise you, that your wife and son will be protected and they will not know they are being protected. Let's go back to my question. Do you really believe your formula works?

Yes, I believe it does! But it involves a tremendous amount of factors and lifestyle changes, especially in your diet. You would have to follow an exact regimen of foods, vitamins, supplements, liquids and exercise. There is also a secret catalyst that triggers the formula which I have not identified as yet, but since the formula appears to work overall, I can always find the catalyst later. Mr. Kelly, what's a catalyst? King Rashid, a catalyst is a special ingredient in a chemical reaction, that allows the reaction to occur. Without it, the reaction could not happen. And even if you tried this entire longevity formula, and it didn't make you younger, you would still become much healthier and live longer with less risk of disease. How are you going to protect my family?

Of the many companies I own, one is a secret service internal protection company, called 'RISS' which stands for 'Rashid International Secret Service'. Many world wide leaders use my agency for their ultimate personal protection. Many are special agents from the FBI, CIA, Secret Service, Israeli Secret Service, U.S. Military Intelligence, Egyptian, Russian KGB, Chinese and Australian Secret Service. They are highly paid and among the best experts available.

The RISS agents are handpicked to work in their respective countries and or where they will 'blend' in. Before and after their 6 month training and without notice they are given truth serum, lie detector testing to make sure they remain loyal. If they become dishonest, they are killed! I have already assigned them to provide protection for your family. They will give you a daily or weekly update if you wish. Yes, I am going to insist that it be done daily.

After a long pause of what's best for Mary and Mike, I had no choice but to accept King Rashid's offer. He said that I would go with him in his car and I would not see my car again. He said to go ahead and remove anything I needed from my car. Together, we would go to the local airport in Knoxville and board his private jet that would take us to West Palm Beach airport. After landing, we would go to his home in West Palm Beach estate where he also had a very large yacht parked. I would be free to stay at the home or leave the coastal area and stay in his yacht. Both places have a full time staff, who are also, 'RISS' agents, who can attend to any needs that I might have, including my protection.

King Rashid, I know you are interested in this formula, as you call it, but can you make the sacrifices it will require, like daily exercise, cutting back on salt to less than 1000-1500 mg/day, and drinking 2 glasses of red wine during the evening meals? I thought alcohol was forbidden in your religion. Mr. Kelly, I own 3 vineyards and if you do go to Dubai someday, you will notice that the city offers everything including some of the finest wines anywhere in the world. And yes, I am willing to do anything to protect my holdings. Now, what do you need to get started?

King Rashid, as for the 'formula' ingredients, I can pick these up probably in one day around West Palm on my own. I will need a new laptop with the latest Microsoft Vista software and a good compatible printer, and a new Palm Treo cell phone. Mr. Kelly, I will get you a new driver's license, new credit cards, new email address, new mail address and various new identification cards and you should select a new name. Also, I will have a new social security number assigned to you. What name would you like? Let's use Ethan Vance. Also, I will need a good acoustical guitar and electronic keyboard. I have been a guitar and piano player for many years and playing these instruments helps me to relax and keeps me motivated and energetic.

Mr. Kelly, you will need a car and you can use one of several parked in the garage. King Rashid, I need to keep my old laptop and cell phone so that I can sync my old information into the new laptop and cell phone. Of course, I will not use old cell phone or laptop email, but they do contain a lot of my research information, especially in the laptop.

Then Mr. Kelly, are we agreed? Yes, but I still want daily and weekly information regarding my wife and son. But what about you, King? What if you refuse to follow the plan I give you? Mr. Kelly, your family will be my first priority and you'll get those daily and weekly reports. I will follow your plan for 30 days and unless I get seriously ill, I will finish it.

The King and I shook hands and as the King's staff returned, he told one of them to drive my car and follow us to the airport. On the way we discussed more details and I asked him to explain how payment was going to happen. Then the King asked, Mr. Kelly, before we leave, is there anything special you need like prescriptions, glasses or anything? You can get new clothes, toiletries and whatever you need in West Palm. Then he said, as for payment, he had already arranged to have ten million dollars deposited in a new account, off shore, in the Bahamas. This bank was an international bank and had many branches throughout the United States. In fact, the name is First Bank of America. He said he would have the bank assign the account under the name I wanted, Ethan Vance, while we are flying to West Palm. After 30 days, if the king is satisfied with my formula and the results, he would than deposit an additional billion dollars. Will that be satisfactory Mr. Kelly? Yes, that will be fine.

About an hour later, we pulled up to the airport area and took a special service road to the private aircraft parking area. There were two pilots doing a pre-flight check outside the big jet. The King said the jet was a Gulf Stream G-500, twin jet with a capacity of 14-19 passengers. The crew included two pilots and one or two attendants. He said the jet cruises about 600 miles per hour and has a range of 6,600 miles. The interior and appointments were incredibly plush.   He also, had a private chef ready to take any meal orders. As we got out of the car, King Rashid said, if there is anything else you need, we can get it at West Palm Beach.

As we entered the aircraft, I was amazed at the lack of security. Don't we have to go through security? No! not on our own aircraft. The jet was unbelievable. It was the most opulent interior I had ever seen on an airplane. In the cockpit, the maze of electronics that was staggering. It looked like a computer room!

After takeoff, King Rashid said he would need to go into his private 'Jet Office' for awhile and set things in motion. He said he was going to introduce me as a new business manager for American operations and that my name would be Mr. Vance. King Rashid, why not introduce me as a health advisor, after all, that's why I am here? Ok, Mr. Vance, that's a good idea.

After the King introduced me to his staff, I began making a list of special activities for the King. After the King finished his phone and computer work, he came out to see if I was ready to discuss the 'schedule'. First, King, are you taking any prescription drugs and what are you taking them for? The King explained that he was on a 'statin' drug to reduce his cholesterol and that he had been taking Hydrodiuril (hydrochlorothiazide) and a beta blocker for his high blood pressure. But his private physician switched him to a newer combination therapy for his high blood pressure. King, is your physician available anytime? Yes, he's my private personal doctor and takes care of my immediate family. He only attends to us. Good, then I suggest you call him and tell him you are considering a new lifestyle diet and rigorous exercise program and therefore, does he have any special instructions for you.

Next, how much do you weigh? And how tall are you? The King said he weighed about 230 pounds and was 5 feet, 10 inches tall. Do you have any other conditions, like for example, diabetes? My last physical exam was last month and my doctor recommended that I should lose 20-30 pounds and that I was a borderline diabetic. Are there any other conditions? King Rashid said no. That was everything as far as he knew.

Now, the next question is critical. How much time can you spend getting started? Because, if you don't start out right and stay with it for at least 30 days, your goals just won't happen and we will both be wasting our precious time. By the way, where can you get your exercise? It must be in private.
Mr. Kelly, excuse me, Mr. Vance, you will have my undivided attention for the next 30 days, except for about 4 hours a day in the afternoon. I need this time to consult with my operation managers, 7 days a week. And my home in West Palm Beach has the latest and finest exercise equipment money can buy.

Ok King, let's go over your new 'schedule'. First, I will need about 2 days to get everything you will need. Also, I will need someone to find and purchase a case of Dragon Green Tea leaves called Long Jing Tea, Zhongguomincha from Hangzhou, China and it must be high grade dragon as well. I doubt if this is available in West Palm. As for everything else, I should be able to purchase in West Palm. The King called in his lead manager and told him to have the tea delivered at his West Palm Beach home by the next day.

King, what I suggest is that as you think of your goal, a new drastic lifestyle adjustment may be necessary. So think in your mind or pretend you have been kidnapped, under guard at all times and that you had to eat only what was offered and had to do what they said. Or, to put in a different way, suppose your plane crashed landed on a deserted island & you had no choice but to eat what was available. Yes, Mr. Vance, I understand what you mean. As the plane descended for the Florida landing, we continued to discuss the 'schedule'. Upon landing, we were met by several guards and quickly left in a large limo.

The King's home was a palace. It was huge and right out of architectural digest magazine. The entire property grounds were heavily guarded, both by well dressed guards and massive electronic security equipment. After meeting all the guards and staff we had a brief late lunch and we made a last minute review of anything needed. King Rashid said he would be tied up until dinner and I said I would be out getting clothes and some things needed for our 'schedule'. He ordered two of his guards to go with me.

After spending some seven hours at Costco, Sams, Fresh Market, Walmart, Publix and Walgreens, nearly every single item required was obtained. I even found some Long Jing Dragon Green Tea at Costco.

At dinner it was decided that the next day, some of his select staff would pick up a new laptop, Palm Treo cell phone, the musical instruments and anything else left on the list. Also, the new 'schedule' was to begin the next morning. The King's personal physician was contacted and it was recommended that he not change any of his medications as yet and the doctor would stay in close contact with the King and check his blood pressure daily and his cholesterol weekly. The next day was the first day on the 'stranded island'.

According to some government public health charts regarding weight/obesity, a person 5 feet, 10 inches tall should weigh around 167-174 pounds. Our immediate goal will be to help you get down 15-20 pounds during the next 30 days.

Kelly's Secret Food Schedule:

Wake up call began with gourmet coffee with non dairy creamer and Nutra-sweet artificial sweetener.

Breakfast:

1. Fiber one cereal-1/2 cup
2. ½ tablespoonful of shelled non-salted walnuts
3. ½ tablespoonful of non-salted almonds
4. ½ tablespoonful of dried cranberries (Craisins)
5. ½ tablespoonful of dried blueberries
6. ½ cup of skim (fat free) milk
7. 1-2 cups of coffee
8. ½ bottle (500 ml bottle) of purified drinking water

Immediately after or up to 30 minutes after breakfast take the following DMVS **(Dietary Minerals, Vitamins and Supplements)** with water:

1. Enteric coated omega-3 fish oil 1000 mg softgel-repeat after lunch.
2. One Calcium with Vitamin D 600 mg tablet
3. 1 and ½ Vitamin C time release 1000 mg caplet
4. 3 Tri-combo 'Move Free' supplement tablets: each tablet contains, Glucosamine Hcl 1500mg, Chondroitin sulfate 200mg, Msm (Methylsulfonylmethane) 1500mg, plus Uniflex extract 250mg and Hyaluronic acid 3.3 mg (joint fluid)
5. One flavored Tums-ex (extra strength) calcium carbonate 750mg

Drink only purified water. This is your breakfast everyday, the rest of your life or until we find something better.

Snack time: 2 hours after breakfast and 2 hours after lunch. Choices:

1-un-salted mini pretzels-Snyder is a popular brand or any other un-salted or low salted (sod=75 mg/20 pretzels or less)
2-or try-Ryvita rye and Oat Bran snacks-very low salt, less than 10mg/serving

3-or try-thin Matzos snack crackers
4-or try-Wasa sourdough bread snack crackers
5-or Mediterranean garlic flavored flatbread
Lunch time: (remember to finish taking any 'DMVS' required after lunch.

After each lunch, have 2-3 cups of hot Long Jing tea and it's recommended to chew some of the leaves, they are extremely healthy.

Monday lunch:

1-Lavasch crackers-garlic flavored or plain sesame (1/2 cup)
2-or sourdough rye Wasa
3-or Ryvita rye and Oat Bran Crispbread and
4-sliced fresh apple
5-sliced raw broccoli
6-sliced raw bell peppers, red are the best
7-serving of mini-size fresh carrots
8-1/2 tablespoonful of 'lite' ranch dressing
9-afternoon tea and leaves

Tuesday lunch:

Same as Monday except-
1-add ½ can of albacore white tuna in water
2-substitute fresh slices of pears in place of apples
3-afternoon tea and leaves

Wednesday lunch:

Same as Monday except-

1-instead of tuna, add 1 and ½ slices of provolone cheese. It should be low in cholesterol, 15 mg per slice or less
2-switch back to slices of fresh apples instead of pears
3-afternoon tea and leaves

Thursday lunch:

Same as Monday
1-afternoon tea

Friday lunch:

Same as Monday except-

1-add ½ can of Atlantic salmon fillet (skinless and boneless); about 3-4 ounces is enough. Or try the tuna again.
2-sustitute fresh sliced pears instead of apples
3-afternoon tea and leaves

This Monday through Friday lunch is semi-permanent. It is extremely healthy, natural, low in cholesterol and contains very little salt.

Saturday lunch:

1-turkey sandwich-try to get fresh turkey from a fresh market type store or meat department. Meat should be baked or broiled. Use olive oil to baste, not butter. The bread choice should be a healthy wheat, rye or multi-grain.
2-fruit, fresh sliced
3-instead of turkey, may substitute chicken, fish (salmon)
4-add some fresh vegetables

Sunday lunch:

Same as Saturday or substitute lunch with 2 scrambled eggs, rye or multi-grain toast, low fat sausage or low fat bacon (cooked in microwave, not fried) or low salt ham. Have toast dry and add some blueberry or strawberry jam. If choose eggs, add pepper and very little salt or no salt. There are several newer egg type products that have no cholesterol and have a good taste.

Late afternoon snacks:

1-Longjing green tea and leaves
2-Gold N Krackle flatbreads-Mediterranean. These are very low sodium, no trans-fats, no preservatives and they are baked.
3-or unsalted fat free mini pretzels
4-or Ryvita rye and Oat Bran whole grain rye Crispbread
5-6-8 ounce glass of Cabernet Sauvignon red wine-sip and drink slowly. This should be served before and during dinner.

Dinners: (between 6:30-8:00pm) General Comments:

1. Serve one bottled water, 500 ml
2. Serve one 6-8 ounce glass of Cabernet Sauvignon red wine. Sip and drink slowly with the main dinner course
3. Dinners should vary. Refrain from processed foods where possible. Such foods may be high in sodium (salt), fats, cholesterol and low in fiber.
4. Choose low fat foods including low fat dressings
5. Breads should be wheat, rye or multi-grain high fiber
6. Use olive oil in place of butter
7. Use as much garlic as you can tolerate
8. Every dinner should include a 'Christmas' vegetable, red or green!
9. Use lots of onions and peppers, green and red
10. Use tomatoes
11. It is recommended that no more than two fish meals be consumed per week. Atlantic fish may be a better choice
12. Substitute turkey, chicken or lean pork
13. 'Reward Meal'-after the first 30 days, have a reward meal, every two weeks for dinner which may include a lean steak and baked fries, or have a cheese pizza with onions and green peppers
14. Main courses:

1-Monday-turkey, fresh, non-processed, baked or broiled

2-Tuesday-shrimp, mussels or scallops or lobster, but cool it on the butter

3-Wednesday-lean pork chops, trim off any fat

4-Thursday-turkey or chicken-lean, no skin

5-Friday-fish-salmon, grouper, tuna, haddock or trout

6-Saturday (every other week)-steak-filet mignon or beef tenderloin very lean

7-Sunday-chicken, turkey, pork-very lean, filets, no skin

Desserts-for the next 30 days:

1-one or two dark chocolate squares with 60-82 % cacao.
2-after 30 days, alternate with chocolate and add no-fat or low fat yogurt 'ice cream'-1/2 serving

This 'Secret' food schedule is to be followed completely for the next 30 days. Then the results will be reviewed.

Pause: King Rashid, before we resume, I want to know how my wife and son are doing! This moment was the most painful I have ever felt, not being with my soul mate and loving partner. I just can't believe I am making the right decision. Am I really protecting my wife &son? There was no news to report yet, except that your wife called the police, and several of her family members, including your family. Several of my 'RISS' agents reported spotting a set of binoculars peering into your house about four houses up the road and also from the deserted island directly across the lake from your house. But after the police were called in, they disappeared. My agents are in control. Do not worry.

You can be sure those binoculars were not for watching birds. Later they were seen driving off after the police showed up. The police were everywhere, all over the neighborhood, and the yacht club and the roads.

It was impossible to concentrate, worrying about my family, but the Kings relentless encouragement to convince me that I was really saving their lives and that made it more bearable.

Kelly's Secret Exercise Schedule: Monday thru Friday

General comments:

1-Plan to spend a minimum of 1 and ½ hours per day of pure exercise between 10:30am-12:30pm. Some folks may have to use a different time schedule. Early morning may be better than late afternoon.

2-Always do some warm-ups before beginning to exercise

3-Always do the cardio exercise first, if possible, it's usually the most difficult. Work hardest to easiest.

4-Legs are about 5 times stronger than arms, do any strong leg exercises first, right after cardio exercises.

5-Drink purified water, about 500 ml during your complete program, but drink small amounts and slowly

6-Have a sweat towel

7-Use a hand sanitizer

8-Set reasonable goals. A reasonable goal of losing 15-20 pounds during the next 30-60 days is possible, if you commit to the entire lifestyle program, including diet.

9-Begin program using the entire 90 minutes, but work lightly and slowly at first. Get used to the 90 minutes.

Special Exercise Schedule:

Treadmill versus the **Elliptical** versus the **Stationary Bicycle**- depending on your knees, your health, what your doctor recommends, a decision should be made based on your ability and physical condition as to how much time you should spend on these machines. The treadmill is considered by many as the most difficult, then the elliptical is considered comparable, but easier on your knees and the stationary bicycle is considered the safest on your legs and joints.

Monday:

1-Treadmill-30 minutes, at 2 up to 2 and ½ mph and flat, no elevation. Walk slowly at first

2-Elliptical-10 minutes, normal resistance and use one with arm handles so that you get full limb movement

3-Stationary bicycle-5 to 10 minutes

4-Stairmaster (stepping machine)-5 minutes (if no Stairmaster, add the 5 minutes to one of the machines above.)

5-Rowing machine-3 minutes (if no rowing machine, add the 3 minutes to one of the machines listed, treadmill, or elliptical, or stationary bike

6-Stationary stretch-5 minutes

Total on machines: 53 minutes

Strength Training Exercise: 37 minutes

1-Abdominal curls-do 12

2-Abdominal curl with twist-do 12

3-Chest press-do 12-Monday, Wednesday, Friday only-gradually increase repetitions each week

4-Shoulder press-do 12-same days and gradually increase repetitions each week

5-Lateral twists-do 20-with exercise neck bar with arms extended

6-Fill in any time left with easy stretches

Tuesday:

1-Exercise machines-same every day for first week, then gradually increase speed and levels each week.

2-Strength training:

A-abdominal exercises-same every day except slowly increase each week

B-biceps-exercise with dumbbells-Tuesday and Thursday only. Gradually increase repetitions each week

Wednesday:

1-Exercise machines-same as Monday

2-Strength training-same as Monday

Thursday:

1-Exercise machines-same as Monday

2-Strength training-same as Tuesday

Friday:

1-Exercise machines-same as Monday

2-Strength training-same as Monday

Remember to drink small amounts of water after any major exercise. And after the exercise session is over, say around 12:30, you should have a regular meal within 30-60 minutes after the session.

Key points:

1-Never exercise alone

2-Develop some activity while exercising like reading a book, or magazine or watching the news. This will help speed up the session.

The King and I worked out together for the entire 4 weeks and it was astonishing to see him so disciplined and determined to conquer his new lifestyle. My daily reports regarding my wife and son were guilt-ridden swords in my heart and brain. Everyday, I thought about quitting and phoning my family. Then one day, it was reported that four men were found shot to death, two at the college campus near where my son was staying and the other two, a few houses down from Mary's house.

The two men at our neighbor's home had apparently killed the neighbors and later the neighbors were found shot to death and discovered at the bottom of the lake in their car. That did it. I knew then, that my decision was the right one. The King told me, that the men that were shot, were most likely agents hired by oldest son, whom he had no respect or faith in. He was ruthless and power hungry and would do anything to take over the King's empire. Next month, when he returns to Dubai, he may finally have to 'do something' with him.

Day 28! Had finally arrived and the King and his staff were truly amazed how good the King looked. He had lost over 25 pounds and his face, still covered with a beard, looked much leaner, his physique looked thinner and his hair looked healthier. He made his latest physician phone call and was given the ok to discontinue his medications. No more lipitor, no more high blood pressure medicine. His doctor was astonished how much weight the King had lost and how much healthier he had become. His cholesterol had dropped to 160.

Day 30! The King called me into his private office. Mr. Vance, I can't tell you how much I respect the wonderful job you did for me. I feel like a new human being. I am healthy again and my energy is back and I look and feel years younger. I owe all to you.

Well thank you King. But you did it. It was nice to see how disciplined and determined you were. Thank you, Mr. Vance. Now let's get back to business. So you say, as long as I continue this 'lifestyle eating and exercise program' that I may live longer and actually get younger? King as far as I know at this point, yes! You have obviously become much healthier, you look better and you look younger. But once you break the chain of antioxidants, vitamins, supplements, drinking of the Long Jing tea, eating and exercising per our plan, the cycle may revert back to normal and normal aging will resume. Are you going to tell me the names of all these and your secret catalyst?

King Rashid, I have prepared for you, enough of a supply to last you a year. Two-four months from today, we should contact each other, and I will give you the secret ingredients if I have identified all of them. The reason is that I still am researching the exact catalyst which generates the body's aging reversal. By that time I will have it isolated. If I find out before that, I will contact you. Will that be satisfactory? Yes, yes, that will be fine. What will you do now, Mr. Vance? The police and FBI are still actively pursuing your disappearance. Your wife and son are doing fine and will be under my continued protection for as long as you wish.

King Rashid, I haven't decided exactly what I am going to do. I believe I will stay out of sight for at least another 6 months. Then everything should have been settled and by then, I will be able to have a handle on just exactly how to control the aging versus reverse aging process.

Mr. Vance, I am leaving tomorrow, and I am going back to Dubai. I am going to gather up my lovely wife and favorite grandchildren and take a long vacation on my other yacht and perhaps enjoy a vacation as I have never done before. Damn! I feel so good. But before I go, I would like to settle our business arrangement.

First the money, one billion dollars, is now being deposited in the banks you requested. A new car is waiting for you, outside. It's in your name and has a built in dvd system that shows you all the features. And as a special bonus, for your great sacrifice, I have purchased you a new home, here in this gated West Palm Beach community. In fact it's only about five or six blocks from here. Also, outside your new home, in the canal, is your new 44 foot yacht. It's completely equipped and it's about the largest boat you can have and run it by yourself, without a crew. Mr. Ramsey, my lead manager will take you over to your new home and boat and spend all the time you need to learn about them. Mr. Ramsey has a master's pilot-charter captain's license and always captains all my yacht trips, among other things. Also, here is your new satellite cell phone. It is programmed to call me directly if you ever need anything. It works anywhere in the world. Oh yes, it's also programmed so that I may call you, if I have any questions.

This is a very special airline card I am giving you. It is called a Premiere First Class Card. It is good on all airlines around the world and you will always fly first class and get the best hotel accommodations, anywhere. So my friend, we can now call each other anytime, from anywhere in the world. I trust you like these bonuses?

King Rashid, I don't know what to say, except, thank you very, very much. We shook hands like two great friends and said our goodbyes, but not for ever.

That afternoon, the King left town and his chief of staff, Mr. Ramsey and I moved my clothes and things over to my new home. The house was gorgeous and big, over 8,000 square feet and the yacht outside was brand new 'Four Winns' Express Cruiser, 44 foot. It had twin IPS (inboard performance system) diesel engines, & over 1,000 total horse power. And it had every option imaginable. I could easily live on it. Mr. Ramsey showed my everything and then gave me the training dvds on the car, the house and the boat. After four hours of training, mostly how to operate and test run the boat, Mr. Ramsey left, but he gave me his private cell number and told me to call him anytime if I needed help or had a question.

The boat was truly amazing. The new 'IPS-Twin Volvo' propulsion system was the state of the art and with the joystick docking system, it was as easy to parallel park as a car. I stayed in the house during the next several weeks. I went out on many boat trips to familiarize myself with ocean boating.

The next two weeks, I spent transferring all my money deposits, except for one off shore, ten million dollar account, to several of my American financial houses, that I used before plus some new ones. I spread the money out, so it didn't stick out so much. A few months later, I purchased a winery in North Carolina, a special ex-military missile silo home not far from Vail, Colorado. I also bought a home in Beaver Creek at Vail, Colorado.

All the time I followed the news about my disappearance and the updates on you, Mary and Mike. At the same time, I kept working with my formula trying to find that darn catalyst that made the aging process reverse. Last month, I found it. By the way, Mary, about four months after I last saw the King, he and all of his close family were all killed after their yacht exploded while they were out to sea. No survivors were ever found. The explosion was so massive, the military was called in to investigate, but the details of what happened were never published.

So Mary, that's the story. I have placed a cooler in your boat. The cooler contains a four months supply of my formula, which works, as you can see. But I know you have a great deal to think about. If you decide to do this, then we need to decide whether to tell Mike. I understand Mike is doing very well, he finished school and is working in Knoxville for one of the largest accounting firms. Mary said he is doing very well and has a serious girl friend and they will probably marry within six months to a year.

Jim, what would I have to do? You would have to leave this place and after it became obvious that you were not aging, but the reverse was happening, you could come and live with me and then we could relive our lives again somewhere private and away from people we know for awhile. You would have to disappear! You can't tell anyone and I mean anyone. It's too risky. We may have to decide not to tell Mike, for his own protection. But Jim, I can't just disappear and leave my family and friends and start all over again. I just can't do it. Mary, I still love you and want us to be together again. But I understand if you say no. Mary broke down and started crying. Mary said, I don't know, I just can't!

Mary, whatever you feel is right, do it. Just think about it. There is a satellite cell phone in the cooler in your boat. You can call me anytime, anywhere in the world. I have set up a special account for you and Mike, of ten million dollars, taxes paid, and to activate your account, just call the special phone number on the plastic card. The instructions are also in your cooler. Mary, you have a lot to ponder, as I have. I can't tell you how much I have missed you, and Mike. Mary, I need to leave now. Mary, I have thought and thought about what I have done and what I need to do now and I have decided, right or wrong, to continue with this aging research and see what I can continue to do to help mankind. I know it sounds corny, but I believe there are many things yet to be discovered and maybe, just maybe I can discover something to help save this reckless world.

They both stood up, hugged each other closely, kissed and as Jim walked away, he turned and said, be careful from now on, don't tell anyone what happened today and trust me and I love you and always will!

Chapter Three: Secret #One-Safeguard The Heart

Perhaps the most important factor in living longer is having a healthy heart. Most experts agree that there are a number of things we can do to 'safeguard' the heart. This chapter will focus on how to make your heart work better and help improve your blood pressure. Be sure to discuss with your doctor, any significant changes in your diet and lifestyle, especially any changes in your weight and blood pressure.

1. Reduce salt (sodium chloride, nacl, sod., or na) intake:

Most Americans eat too much salt each day. Some experts feel that this one factor, too much sodium per day, may be the leading contributor to high blood pressure, especially in later years of life. Most folks eat between 2,300 to 4,700mg (milligrams) a day. (1,000mg=1 gram) recommended daily dose is 1,500mg for adults and even less for older adults. Some even recommend as little as 500mg/day.

One of the main sources of sodium (salt) excess is 'processed foods' with salt added and sodium containing additives. Nearly 80% of our sodium intake may come from processed foods. Start checking labels when grocery shopping, especially with processed meats, dinners, frozen foods and canned foods. For example: a teriyaki chicken, plain, serving size of ¾ cup may contain 2,190 mg of sodium salt. That's just one meal. A frozen chicken fingers meal may contain 1070 mg of sodium salt. Having ham for breakfast, just 4 ounces, may contain 3,045 mg of sodium. A can of Chef Boyardee beef ravioli, one cup, may contain 1,120 mg of sodium.

One beef pot pie may contain 1,000 mg of sodium. Pretzel sticks, just 2 ounces, may contain 1,029mg of sodium. One take out submarine sandwich with salami, cheese and vegetable may contain 1,650mg of sodium salt. One cup of chicken noodle soup may contain 1,107 mg of sodium. Just one package of ramen noodles, beef, may contain 1,236mg of salt.

Spanish food, take out nachos with cheese, beans, ground beef, and peppers may contain 1,800mg of sodium per serving size. Applebee's burger with fries, one serving, may contain 2,713 mg of sodium salt. Denny's 'All American Grand Slam', one serving may contain 1,826mg of sodium. Denny's buffalo wings, 12, may contain a whopping 5,552 mg of sodium.

KFC extra crispy chicken breast, may contain 1,230 mg of sodium. One McDonald's bagel, steak egg and cheese, may contain 1,540mg of sodium. Panera Bread sierra turkey sandwich may contain 2,320mg of sodium. Quizno's sub-turkey lite may contain 1,909 mg of sodium. Wendy's big bacon classic may have 1,460 mg of sodium. Obviously, salt may improve flavor, help in some preservation of foods, but common sense and caution should be used to reduce excess consumption.

(See Chapter four: Counter Chart-Secret #Three, for a more extensive food and restaurant review of sodium, calories, protein, fats, cholesterol, carbohydrates, and fiber)

Kelly's Recommendations:

1-Meats-seek out more 'fresh' meats that have not been 'processed'

2-Check labels on salt or sodium contents

3-Eat more fresh vegetables and fruits which have either no sodium or very little.

4-Eating out can be a good experience, try eating less, eat slower and add more vegetables and fruits.

5-Try splitting your meals or eat less and take the rest home for another meal.

6-Excess sodium may be the greatest cause of high blood pressure, especially in America, and can easily be improved by you.

7-Drink more purified water. Don't drink tap water. Remember one gallon of purified water can cost less than a can of soda pop.

Some experts say, adults aged 19-50 should get no more than 1,500 mg of sodium per day. Those folks between 50-70 should get 1,300mg/day and folks over 70, 1,200mg/day. The upper limit should not go beyond 2,300mg/day.

What does Sodium do?

Sodium regulates your body's fluid level, both inside and outside your cells. This monitors your blood volume, blood pressure and the acidity of your body. The movement of sodium into and out of your cells allows other important substances to make this journey too, helping to transmit nerve impulses and electrical messages vital to your body's minute-to-minute functioning.

Most people associate too much salt with high blood pressure. This assumption has been proven by studies done worldwide. In places where little salt is used, blood pressure does not go up with age as it does in the United States. Reducing salt intake, can lower your blood pressure in people who have it, and even to a lesser degree, in people who have normal blood pressure.

About 10-15% of all people with high blood pressure are very sensitive to salt. If they reduce the amount of salt they eat, their blood pressure goes down. People who are not salt sensitive, will not see such a dramatic downward trend, but their blood pressure will still go down. It's wise to eat less salt because keeping your blood pressure values within normal range reduces your risk of heart attacks, strokes, and kidney disease.

When people are told to eat less salt, most stop or reduce salting their food at the table. That may not be the best approach. Daily sodium intake doesn't come from salt added while cooking or eating. That equals to a little more than 10% of your daily intake. Foods may contain another 10% naturally and then that leaves the vast majority, nearly 80% coming from salts added and sodium containing additives or processed foods, especially American foods.

2. Cholesterol (chol):

Good cholesterol intake, ideally, is less than 200 mg/dl (deciliter) per day.

Why is cholesterol so important?

Basically, cholesterol serves many vital functions:

1-Converts into Vitamin D and enhances the absorption of calcium.

2-Part of bile salts which digest fats

3-Cholesterol is converted into sex hormones, estrogen, progesterone and testosterone.

4-Converts into Aldosterone which is part of a complex system that regulates blood volume, blood pressure and mineral balance.

5-Cholesterol is converted into all the stress hormones, including Cortisol, Cortisone, and Corticosterone.

6-Cholesterol is present in every cell membrane and pliability determines what moves in and out of every cell, every moment, every day, every year.

7-Cholesterol coats plaque laid down in blood vessels, and acts like a bandaid, covers any irritation, any inflammation and protects it from getting larger.

8-Cholesterol insulates nerve cells and helps skin cells retain moisture.

9-Cholesterol makes up a major part of your brain.

10-Cholesterol is a white, waxy fat-like substance.

11-Having too much cholesterol in your blood is not healthy. Excess can be deposited onto your artery walls, narrowing them and interfering with normal blood flow.

You get cholesterol every time you eat animal foods, such as meat, poultry, fish, eggs, milk, yogurt, cheese, or butter. There is no cholesterol in foods that grow in the ground. Vegetables, fruits, nuts, seeds, cereals, and grains have none. Cholesterol can also be made in the body. In fact, most people make 3 times more cholesterol than they eat in their foods.

On the average, American men eat about 330 mg of cholesterol per day. Women eat about 240 mg per day. The federal government's National Cholesterol Education Program recommends no more than 200 mg/day. The American Heart Association (aha) recommends that you limit cholesterol to less than 300 mg/day and 200 mg/day if you already have heart disease.

Cholesterol is made in the body, mostly by the liver and makes about 800-1500 mg/ day. Normal cholesterol intake should be 200mg/day. HDL=high density lipoprotein is good cholesterol (less than 40 is good). LDL=low density lipoprotein is bad cholesterol (lower than 160 is better).

16 ways to lower Cholesterol:

1-Take Alpha Lipoic Acid-dietary supplement and antioxidant, improves cellular redox state by scavenging reactive oxygen species.

2-Eat more artichokes-lowers blood cholesterol.

3-Use Curcumin (aka-turmeric)-anti-inflammatory, anti-tumor and antioxidant.

4-Drink Green Tea (including decaffeinated)-improves bad cholesterol by lowering LDL, and anti-tumor.

5-Consume more fish oils-help regulate cholesterol because of high levels of omega-3.

6-Consume more garlic-helps prevent heart disease by reducing atherosclerosis (hardening of the arteries),high cholesterol and high blood pressure.

7-Use more ginger-reduces inflammation, helps thin blood and lowers cholesterol.

8-Consume grapefruit pectin-helps reduce cholesterol.

9-Use Gugulipid-helps lower cholesterol.

10-Use olive oil leaf extract-herbal antioxidant, helps reduce LDL (bad cholesterol).

11-Use Perilla oil-rich in omega-3 and therefore helps regulate cholesterol.

12-Eat more soy-help reduce cholesterol

13-Use Policosanol-lowers LDL and raises HDL and helps prevent atherosclerosis.

14-Take Vitamin E-antioxidant and helps prevent heart disease by lowering LDL

15-Use Tocotrienols (more Vitamin E family)-lowers LDL.

16-Check testosterone levels-testosterone is derived from cholesterol.

One Japanese study stated a 'quick fix for cholesterol reduction': take 1 cup of broccoli sprouts/day for 1 week. The 3 day old broccoli plant contains high concentrations of a potential antioxidant previously shown to help prevent stomach ulcers and several types of cancer and other diseases.

Check **Chapter Five: Secret # Three-Counter Chart,** for review of foods and food preparations for cholesterol comparisons. Listed below, are some eye opening cholesterol contents: note: the serving size may not be accurate for some folks who may be bigger eaters. But the size is average.

Teriyaki chicken plain 6 ounce=92 mg
Canadian bacon grilled 6 ounce=81 mg
Cheddar cheese 1 ounce=30 mg
Beef brisket 3 ounce=81mg
Chicken broiled breast 4.9 ounce=119mg
Boneless skinless chicken breasts 3 ounce=70mg
Chicken fingers meal 7.1 ounce=70mg
Egg deviled 2 halves=280mg
Eggnog 1 cup=149mg
French toast w/butter 2 slices=116mg
Turkey giblets 1 cup=606mg
Ham center slice 4 ounce=80mg
Hamburger double w/bacon/cheese 1=110mg
Corn dog 1=79mg
Hot dog beef 2 ounce=35mg
Liver pan fried 3 ounce=410mg

Pecan pie 1 slice=65mg
Pork roast au jus 5 ounce=85mg
Salmon cake 3 ounce=104mg
Deep fried calamari 1 serv=423mg
Trout baked 3 ounce=63mg
Tuna chunk light in water 2 ounce=30mg
Turkey leg w/skin roasted 1.2 pounds=466mg
Applebee's burger w/fries 1 serv=263mg
Bob Evans country biscuit breakfast 1 serv=267mg
Boston Market ½ chicken w/skin 9.7 ounce=280mg
Denny's All American Slam 1 serv=828mg
Denny's senior omelete 1 serv=515mg
Jack In The Box breakfast croissant sausage 1=240mg
KFC extra crispy breast 1=135mg
McDonald's bagel steak, egg and cheese 8.5 ounce=265mg
McDonald's big breakfast 9.4 ounce=455mg
McDonald's egg mcmuffin 4.9 ounce=235mg
What-A-Burger biscuit w/bacon, egg and cheese 1=252mg

More ways to 'Safeguard Your Heart'

There is growing evidence that atherosclerosis or hardening of the arteries results from, in part, chronic low-grade **inflammation.** The state of continuous inflammation may contribute to the development of **plaques** on the artery walls. There is strong evidence that when patients already have some plaque build-up as we all do by the age of 50. The immune system perceives this as an injury, sparking more inflammation. Then the white blood cells that are involved in the inflammatory response, attack the plaque, says Dr. Robert Bonow. In doing so, the plaque can rupture, initiating a blood clot. This may explain why ½ of all strokes and heart attacks occur in people with normal or even lower cholesterol.

People with high inflammation, but low cholesterol have a worse survival rate than those with high cholesterol and low inflammation. There is a simple test called **'CRP'** (c reactive protein). The 'C' Reactive Protein is a molecule produced by the liver in response to an inflammatory signal. An increased reading may triple the risk of heart attack.

How to low 'CRP' levels:

1-Brush and floss:

There is a direct link between gum disease and tooth loss with higher risk of atherosclerosis and higher CRP levels. One study even suggests that cavities, gingivitis and missing teeth are stronger predictors of cardiovascular problems. Bacteria that cause these ailments in the mouth can appear in the same atherosclerotic plaque associated with cardiovascular disease, per Michael Rethman, DDS. One theory is that bacteria enter the bloodstream directly through the inflamed gum tissues.

2-Stop smoking:

When you smoke a cigarette, over 1000 chemicals enter your body, many of them irritants that get into the blood stream, triggering an inflammatory response. Smoking is especially inflammatory to an artery's endothelium, its interior lining. Because each cigarette adds new damage, the blood vessels never have time to heal, making them magnets for fatty plaque. 'Butting out' the habit, immediately reduces inflammation and eventually reduces the risk of cardiovascular disease back to levels of non-smokers

3-Banish the belly fat:

Any excess poundage is a possible inflammation inducer, because fat cells are a virtual factory for producing inflammatory molecules. But belly fat is particularly dangerous. Fat tissue inside the abdominal cavity is especially metabolically active because it secretes even more harmful proteins into the blood stream, so says Dr. Bonow. In one recent study, women ages 50-70 whose waist is larger than 35 inches, also had lower levels of a specific inflammation fighting hormone. This is another great reason to daily exercise program and help burn excess calories and fat. For example to burn about 500 calories, you would need to walk about 5 miles.

4-Rethink your diet and lifestyle eating:

Fatty, cholesterol laden foods clog your arteries. White bread, baked potatoes, and other foods with high glycemic index (foods that are digested and converted to glucose most quickly) can harm, by contributing to inflammation by causing quick, dramatic spikes in blood sugar and increasing the **production of free radicals** that damage cells and trigger inflammation. But here are some 'good guys food' that fight inflammation: omega-3 fatty acids-olive oil, walnuts, and cold water fish such as salmon, mackerel and herring. One study showed that **1,000 mg of fish-oil caps per day** can lower the risk of sudden cardiac death by nearly half.

Plant foods rich in certain disease-fighting natural chemicals may also have potent anti-inflammatory effect. Tomatoes, blueberries, eggplant and fiber-rich grains for optimal heart health and choose whole grains over white flour. Also, eating smaller and more frequent meals causes a slower spike in blood glucose and therefore, less inflammation.

5-Stay in for lunch:

Long term exposure to air pollution, especially from car exhaust and coal-fired power plants, pose a greater risk of death from heart disease than from respiratory ailments. Air pollution provokes inflammation and accelerates atherosclerosis.

6-Control your emotions and stress:

Anxious or depressed folks have higher rates of heart disease. Some studies find they have higher rates of inflammation, whether stress causes inflammation is still debatable. But it is well established that cortisol, adrenaline and other stress related substances damage the endothelium, possible contributing to the development of atherosclerosis. Meditation and other stress-managed strategies, help reduce inflammation, especially with a heart-healthy diet. Also, exercise, laughter, having pets, help relax blood vessels and improve blood flow.

7-Red wine grapes:

Many studies recommend red wine for its antioxidant, heart-helping abilities. But drink only in moderation. Too much, can be worse for you than no drinking at all. There may be some connection between too much drinking and inflammation and heart disease.

Comments about good medicine:

Non-steroidal anti-inflammatory drugs ('NSAIDS') may seem an obvious way to lower inflammation, but recent history shows that drugs such a Vioxx may present their own cardiovascular dangers. Even some 'OTC' (over the counter, non-prescription) pain relievers may raise the risk of a heart attack. Check with your doctor and pharmacist. Some statins, that help lower cholesterol, like Lipitor, Zocor, Mevacor and Crestor may improve crp levels in as little as 2 weeks. There are a virtual multitude of prescription drugs that help reduce crp levels, cholesterol and inflammation, so check with your doctor for what's best for you.

How To Lower Your Blood Pressure:

Never stop your prescription medications without checking with your doctor and pharmacist. Listed below are some alternative methods used by some to assist in lower blood pressure.

1-Reduce salt (sodium) intake to less than 1,500-2,000mg/day. Note: it's the chloride portion of the sodium chloride that causes the high blood pressure, not the sodium.

2-Lose weight.

3-Reduce stress-slow down-relax.

4-Eat more frequently, 5-6 times per day, but in smaller portions.

5-Lower alcohol consumption-it increases blood pressure by triggering production of anti-diuretic hormone and depletes the body of potassium and magnesium.

6-Exercise regularly.

7-Consume 5-9 servings of fruits and vegetables daily. We need potassium and magnesium from fruits to keep blood pressure normal. Potassium helps flush out excess salts and water. Magnesium helps the blood vessels relax.

8-Include calcium containing foods or supplements.

9-Decrease saturated fats especially from cheeses, processed meats and lard.

10-Increase mono-unsaturates such as olive oil, canola oil, omega-3 fatty acids.

11-Cut back on your intake of high sodium foods, like cheese, crackers, processed meats like bacon, bologna, corned beef, ham, hot dogs, salami and ethnic foods like Chinese, Italian, Japanese and Mexican. Cut back on frozen dinners, high salt snack crackers, pickles, popcorn, potato chips, pretzels, salad dressings, salted nuts and soy sauce.

12-Use more natural herbs when cooking.

13-Use more pepper and less salt.

14-Use more mustard and less mayonnaise.

15-Eat more garlic.

16-Drink more green tea.

More Heart Health Factors:

1-Lifestyle, not heredity is the biggest culprit. High cholesterol quadruples the risk of heart attack.

2-Diabetes is especially deadly for women, quadrupling their Risk of heart attack, for men it doubles. Like smoking, diabetes causes platelets to stick together, resulting in scores of tiny clots. These clots clog the microscopic blood vessels that feed nerves and arteries, which is the key reason diabetes destroys circulation.

3-Psychological stress, stressful life events, behavioral disorders and depression nearly triple heart attack risk. Depressed people with heart disease are 4 times more likely to have a heart attack or die.

4-Abdominal obesity doubles heart attack risk in men and women.

5-High blood pressure nearly triples a man's risk of having a heart attack and more than doubles heart attack risk for women. Narrowed blood vessels force the heart to work harder, slowly wearing it out.

6-Smokers are 2-3 times more likely to have a heart attack than non-smokers. Cigarette smoke damages the artery walls, and paving the way for inflammation and cholesterol build up.

7-Alcohol is another platelet blocker. In modest amounts alcohol reduces the risk of a man's heart attack by 12 % and by 60% on women. All forms of alcohol help in small amounts. Too much beer, or hard liquor, more than 2 per day can promote heart disease, cancer and alcoholism.

8-Eating fruits and vegetables daily can cut the risk of heart attack by 30-40%. They lower the bad cholesterol, improve blood sugar and replace foods that might not be as healthy.

9-Exercise, even moderate, reduces a man's heart attack risk by 23% and a woman's by 46%. Even a nice walk in the park can improve cholesterol, help reduce tendency towards diabetes, improve blood sugar and promote blood vessel growth. Regular exercise is the key

Chapter Four: Eating Review-Kelly's Secret #Two

"Give me a double cheeseburger with mayo and bacon and large fries, but since I am on a diet, give me a large 'diet coke'".

Some folks say, tell me what you eat and I'll tell you what you are. But most will agree, that what you eat determines how long and how well you will live.

Lifestyle is the dominant factor in good health and even more important in longevity. Heredity is important but perhaps not as much as what you do and what you eat. Most fad type diets do not last after a period of time. Many researchers suggest a change of lifestyle, such as eating foods with less fat, less salt, less cholesterol, more fiber, less calories, less carbohydrates, and proper protein. They also recommend a steady exercise program of at least 30 minutes a day, 5 days a week. Many other factors are also important such as giving up smoking, moderate alcohol consumption and controlling stress are also very important.

This chapter will start off with a trip to the food store, and make a beginning list of foods to try. Then each eating category-Calories, Protein, Fat, Carbohydrates, and Fiber will be reviewed as well as Sodium and Cholesterol which we have already covered in the previous chapter, 'Safeguard The Heart'.

Trip To The Food Store: (General Comments):

1. Cereals-high fiber cereals, such as Fiber One, Bran Buds, All-Bran Extra Fiber, 100% Bran, Grape Nuts, Natural Bran Flakes, Cracklin Oat Bran, Bran Chex, and Raisin Bran-Rp, and others contain substantial amounts of important fiber. Cereals are important, because a good cereal breakfast should be enjoyed everyday of your life.

In fact, adding some banana slices, blueberries, walnuts, almonds, and cranberries to a high fiber cereal is an extremely healthy meal. Special note: adults should only use skim or fat free milk; it has very little fat, less cholesterol and more calcium.

2. Fruits and vegetables-make it happen, pick your favorites, but bananas, blueberries, apples, pears, red and green peppers, onions, garlic, celery, broccoli, carrots, spinach, acorn squash, pole beans, sweet potatoes and many others, offer an excellent source of very healthy foods as well as reducing the risk of disease. Some studies recommend vegetables that are more red, like tomatoes and red peppers have more anti-cancer properties. Seasoning is ok, especially with pepper and herbs, but back off from excess salt. Try reduced fat salad dressings and use more olive oil, lower fat mixes and balsamic vinegars. Fruits and vegetables are also excellent snack items with no cholesterol, no fat, and no salt.

3. Meats and fish-try to avoid 'processed' meats and fish. They may be loaded with sodium and sodium additives. Ask for fresh cuts of meats, poultry and fish. Turkey is considered by many, one of the more healthy meats, because it generally is more lean (white meat) and has less fat than most red meats. In order of most healthy (by some studies):

(1)Fish-salmon, trout, tuna, mackerel, cod (especially the Atlantic fish) and many other favorites are considered healthier because (when they are fresh) they contain minimum amounts of salt, no sugars, smaller amounts of bad cholesterol, less fat, more protein and also contain solid amounts of omega-3 fish oil (fatty acids-Epa[eicosapentaenoic acid], and Dha [docosahexaenoic acid].These acids are notorious for improving cholesterol and fighting cardiovascular inflammation.

(2) Turkey, chicken, lean pork chops, and then red meats do contain important proteins, calories, and fats, but they also may contain some excess of cholesterol and sodium and practically zero fiber. People who 'must have meat' with every meal may tend to develop excessive cholesterol, higher blood pressure and may risk cardio-vascular problems.

It can be more healthful to balance food groups. Most experts agree that too much red meat can be harmful. Eat more turkey, or chicken or lean pork or lower cholesterol cheeses. Below is a comparison of popular choices and serving sizes (which are likely smaller than some may think they require) and also listed are things you should look for.

Serving size-Calories-Protein-Fat-Cholesterol-Carbohydrates-Fiber-Sodium(sod):**Calories are measured as an amount of 'fuel' or standard of energy. Fat is listed as grams (gm). Cholesterol is measured in milligrams, carbohydrates are measured in grams. Fiber is measured in grams. Protein is measured in grams and Sodium (sod) is measured in milligrams (mg).**

1-Turkey w/o skin, roasted-4 oz-cal 183/prot 35/fat 4/chol 81/carb 0/fib 0/sodium (sod or na) 75

2-Tuna light in water-3 oz-cal 60/prot 13/ fat 1/chol 30/ carb 0/fib 0/ sod 250

3-Snapper 3 oz-cal 109/prot 22/fat 1/chol 40/carb 0/ fib 0/sod 48

4-Salmon 3 oz-cal 155/prot 22/ fat 7/ chol 60/carb 0/fib 0/sod 48

5-Pork tenderloin, fresh lean roasted 3 oz-cal 139/prot 24/fat 4/ chol 67/carb 0/fib 0/ sod 48

6-Hot dog beef 2 oz-cal 180/prot 7/fat 16/chol 35/carb 1/fib 0/ sod 585

7-Hamburger double patty w bacon/cheese 1 serv-cal 457/prot 28/ fat 28/chol 110/carb 22/fib 0/ sod 635

8-Cod Atlantic fresh 3 oz-cal 89/prot 19/fat 1/ chol 47/carb 0/fib 0/sod 66

9-Beef tenderloin 3 0z-cal 194/prot 23/fat 11/cho 72/carb 0/fib 0/sod 52

10-Chicken skinless breasts 3 oz-cal 110/prot 25/fat 2/chol 70/ carb 0/fib 0/sod 30

11-Cheese cheddar low fat 1 oz-cal 49/prot 9/fat 2/chol 6/carb 1/fib 0/sod 174

12-Egg 1-cal 75/prot 6/fat 5/chol 213/carb 1/fib 0/sod 63

Now compare w/vegetables and fruits:

1-Celery fresh 1.3 oz-cal 6/prot 0/fat 0/ chol 0/ carb 1/fib 1/sod 35

2-Broccoli raw chopped ½ cup-cal 12/prot 1/fat 0/chol 0/carb 2/ fib 1/sod 12

3-Apple 1-cal 81/prot 0/fat 0/chol 0/ carb 21/fib 2/sod 0

4-Blueberries 1 cup-cal 82/prot 1/fat 1/chol 0/carb 20/fib 0/sod 9

5-Banana 1-cal 109/prot 1/fat 0/chol 0/carb 28/fib 3/sod 1

A quick glance shows an immense difference in calories, protein, fat, cholesterol, fiber, carbohydrates and sodium contents between vegetables and fruits and meats, fish and eggs. Also, eggs are a great source of protein, calories and low fat, but the high cholesterol contents, usually around 100mg or more per egg make them potentially harmful if consumed in excess or too frequently.

There are many 'egg' products now available without or minimal amounts of cholesterol.

4. Cheeses- Cheeses are a good source of food instead of meats. However, many may contain significant amounts of cholesterol, fat and salt. Guard against excess and too much frequency. They are also an excellent source of calories, protein and moderate fat. Yogurts are also a good meat substitute and usually have less calories, less cholesterol, less fat and less salt. Here are some popular cheeses to review:

American cheese 1 oz-cal 93/prot 6/fat 7/chol 18/carb 2 fib 0/sod 337

Cheddar cheese 1 oz-cal 114/prot 7/fat 9/chol 30/carb 0/fib 0/sod 230

Cheddar low fat 1 oz-cal 49/prot 9/fat 2/chol 6/carb 1/fib 0/sod 174

Mozzarella cheese 1 oz-cal 80/prot 6/fat 6/chol 22/carb 1/fib 0/sod 106

Provolone cheese 1 oz-cal 100/prot 7/fat 8/chol 20/carb 1/fib 0/sod 248

Swiss cheese 1 oz-cal 107/prot 8/fat 8/chol 26/carb 1/fib 0/sod 74

Yogurt cheese 1 oz-cal 80/prot 6/fat 7/chol 15/carb 0/fib 0/sod 60

American w/jalapeno pepper 1 oz-cal 80/prot 6/fat 6/chol 20/carb 2/fib 1/sod 260

Muenster cheese 1 oz-cal 100/prot 6/fat 8/chol 25/carb 0/fib 0/sod 140

Parmesan cheese 1 oz-cal 40/prot 4/fat 3/chol 10/carb 0/fib 0/sod 240

Many 'low fat' cheeses now have improved flavor and may serve as a better health source.

5. Milk-

Most experts advise drinking some milk daily, but the main suggestion for adults is fat free or skim milk. One cup contains only 90 calories, has 8 grams of protein, contains little or no fat, has only 5 mg of cholesterol and 11 gms of carbohydrates. Drinking one cup a day should provide about 30% of the daily required calcium and about 25% of daily needed Vitamin D. Overall, milk can be an excellent supplement to help good bone development and maintenance.

6. Snacks-

Most Americans love their snacks. It's very easy to overdo it. Seek out snacks with reduced fat and lower salt content. Here are only a few for comparison:

Cheez-Its w/40 % less fat, 29 pieces-cal 130/prot 4/fat 4/chol 0/carb 20/fib 1/sod 360

Triscuits reduced fat 1/3 less 7 pieces-cal 120/prot 3/chol 0/carb 21/fib 3/sod 160

Ruffles light ½ cal and fat free 15 pieces-cal 75/prot 3/fat 0/chol 0/carb 16/fib 1/sod 230

Snyders pretzels fat free nibblers 16 pieces-cal 120/prot 3/fat 0/chol 0/carb 25/fib 1/sod 200

The low fat snacks listed above contain more than one ounce of quantity and still contain less fat

Now compare some of the similar snacks that are not low in fat or salt. 'baked' versus fried snacks usually have less fat.

Doritos regular 1 oz-cal 140/prot 2/fat 7/chol 0/carb 18/fib 1/sod 120

Fritos king size 1 oz-cal 150/prot 2/fat 9/chol 0/carb 16/fib 1/sod 180

Pringles original 1 oz-cal 160/prot 2/fat 11/chol 0/carb 15/fib 1/sod 170

Oreo cookies 3 pieces-cal 160/prot 1/fat 7/chol 0/carb 23/sod 222

There are many snacks which are considered more healthy. Here are a few popular choices:

Ryvita Rye and Oat Bran serving-cal 35/prot 1/fat 0/chol 0/fib 2/carb 8/sod 10

Gold D'N Krackle Flatbreads ½ oz-cal 58/prot 2/fat 1/chol 0/carb 11/fib 0/sod 15

Wasa Fiber Rye serving-cal 30/prot 1/fat 1/2/chol 0/carb 7/fib 2/sod 50

Lavasch crackers ½ oz-cal 60/prot 2/fat 2/chol 0/carb 10/fib 1/sod 65

Manischewitz thin matzos unsalted serving-cal 90/prot 2/fat 0/chol 0/carb 20/fib 0/sod 0

The healthiest of all snacks are fruits. Most natural fruits contain no fat, no cholesterol and no salt.

7. Seasonings and oils-

Many people enjoy salads and feel that they are a good healthy food supplement and that can be true. But, if the salad is 'flooded' with high fat, high cholesterol, and high sodium, it may not be so healthy.

There are many dressings with improved taste, and lower fat. Most of the popular favorites come in lighter and even no fat flavors. Olive oil, a mono-unsaturated fatty acid, is considered by most, the oil of choice. Olive oil contains an ingredient, oleocanthal, which works even as a pain killer the same way the drug ibuprofen works to suppress pain. The anti-inflammatory properties of oleocanthal, may help explain the reduced incidence of certain cancers, stroke and heart disease especially in the Mediterranean populations that use large amounts of olive oil in their diets.

Mayonnaise, a very popular dressing, may contain 100 calories per tablespoonful, and 11 gms of fat, 5 mg of cholesterol and 75 mg of sodium. 'Light' 'mayo' still retains good flavor, but contains about ½ the fat and calories of regular mayonnaise. Mustard is recommended to use in place of mayo, where possible, especially on hamburgers, hot dogs, sandwiches, meats, cheeses, because one teaspoonful, contains zero calories, zero fat, zero cholesterol, zero carbohydrates and only 55 mg of sodium.

8. Breads-

There are many types of breads. Many breads are a good source of food in general, and many contain good fiber, calories and carbohydrates as well as protein. Many experts recommend multi-grain breads as a good all around bread source. Regular white bread is one of the lesser healthy breads. Bagels are also considered a better source of nutrition than white breads because they are higher in protein, lower in carbohydrates, higher in fiber and higher in calories. But they may also contain more fat and sodium .

A balanced approach to eating breads may be more healthy. Breads are starches and after the body converts what it needs for energy, excess starch is converted and stored as fat. Use more wheat and multigrain breads.

9. Desserts-

Desserts, other than fresh fruits, are generally loaded with sugar & often contain fat, sodium, little or no fiber, lots of calories and carbohydrates and very little if any, protein.

1-Ice cream is a delightful dessert, but it is not very healthy. For example, ½ cup may contain-cal 130/prot 2/fat 7/chol 25/carb 16/ fib 0/sod 45. Switching to a low fat light yogurt 'ice cream', which may taste just like ice cream, can be a wise move.

2-Low fat light yogurt ½ cup-cal 130/prot 4/fat 3/chol 10/carb 24/fib 0/sod 105.

3-Chocolate Ghirardelli squares 60 % cacao dark chocolate is a popular type of dessert. It is interesting, because not only is it a tasty treat, it is also considered a healthy antioxidant food source. Dark chocolate and especially 60% or higher cacao is recommended by many as aid to longevity. Generally, 2 squares contain-cal 110/prot 1/fat 8.5/chol 0/carb 11.5/fib 1.5/sod 0.

How Much Should You Weigh?

Most Americans are overweight and a growing number of those are obese. Obesity leads may lead to increased risks of diseases like diabetes, heart disease, cancer, high blood pressure just to name a few.

Let's review one example and see how you compare. Then we will review how to figure out where you fit in and where you should fit in.

For example:

An average person, 5 feet, 10 inches tall with a 'BMI'(body mass index) of 24 should weigh about 167 pounds. Another person, say 5 feet, 5 inches tall with a BMI of 22, should weigh about 132 pounds. Remember this book is mainly aimed at adults, and particularly, older adults.

What is 'BMI'?

BMI, is a simple math calculation used to determine your body mass index. BMI takes into account height and weight and measures fat tissue to separate out the weight of muscle and the skeleton.

How do you find your BMI?

Divide your weight, in pounds, by your height, in inches, squared and multiply by 703. For example, if you are 6 feet (72 inches) tall and weigh 190 pounds, your BMI is 25.8 the calculation is 190 divided by 5,184 (that's 72x72), multiplied by 703.

What BMI is considered a healthy range?

A normal BMI range is 18.5 to 24.9. Lower is considered underweight. Overweight is 25 to 29.9 and more than 30 is considered obese. So the person in the example above can move into the normal recommended range by losing about 5 to 6 pounds.

Is it possible to have a high BMI and not be fat?

Yes, it's possible, especially with muscular athletes who are in very good condition. Some folks in the 25 to 29.9 range may not have excess body fat, but many more do. And most people in the obese range are carrying around levels of excess fat that put them at risk.

What are Calories? What is Fat? What is Fiber? What is Protein? And what are Carbohydrates?

1. Calories (cal):

Calories are calories, whether they come from chocolate or pears. All foods, except water, have some calories. Whenever you eat, you take in calories. You body is like a machine that uses food calories as 'fuel'. When the amount of fuel you take in equals the amount of fuel you need for your body to run, your weight should remain constant. If you eat too many calories, and your body uses only what it needs, then it stores the excess calories, for future use. Common storage areas are your thighs, hips and waist. If you eat too few calories, your body will draw on its fuel reserves and your thighs, hips and waist will get slimmer as the surplus is depleted.

Calories come from fat, protein, and carbohydrates in foods. Fat has the most calories of the three. It has more than twice as many as proteins and carbohydrates. For example: one teaspoonful of 'fat' equals 40 calories, while a teaspoonful of either carbohydrate or protein has only 16 calories.

If you cut the calories, you will lose weight. If you eat too many calories, even from healthy foods, you gain weight.
It doesn't matter if those calories come from bread, high protein meat or mayonnaise. The key to long term weight control is to burn as many as you eat.

In a recent government survey, the average man eats 2,550 calories per day and the average woman eats 1,850 calories per day.

2. Fat:

Fat has a bad reputation that is undeserved. It is important for providing energy, supplying essential fatty acids that the body cannot make, insulating the body, protects vital organs, stores fat-soluble vitamins, and is part of all cell membranes. And fat also makes some foods taste good.

Fats or 'lipids' as some scientists call them, represent a large family of several substances. You get fats from the foods you eat, and your body can also make some fats. Food fats are made up of strands of 'fatty acids'. Think of these fatty acids as strands of beads that vary in combination and the number of beads depending on their chemical combination.

There are three main types of fatty acids:

1-Saturated

2-Mono-unsaturated

3-Polyunsaturated.

Many foods contain combinations of all three fatty acids, but we label foods as sources of saturated (butter), monounsaturated (olive oil) or polyunsaturated (corn oil) based on the predominated fat in the food. It has been recently suggested that the 'type' of fat you eat may be more important than the amount of fat you eat.

Some experts recommend that your daily fat intake make up 20-35% of your total calories. This means that if you regularly eat 1,800 calories per day, somewhere between 360-630 calories should come from fat.

Even though a moderate fat intake may be healthy, it doesn't mean that a high fat intake is in any way good for you. In a recent study, it was found that 'dieters' who were given 35% of their daily calories as fat, found it easier to stick with their weight loss program and kept the weight off longer.

What are Trans-Fats?

Trans-fats or trans-fatty acids (trans-fats) are a type of unsaturated fat and may be monounsaturated or polyunsaturated. They occur in small quantities in meats and dairy products from ruminants (hoofed animals). Most trans-fats consumed today, are industrially created as a side effect of partial 'hydrogenation' of plant oils. Partial hydrogenation changes a fat's molecular structure raising the melting point and reducing rancidity.

Unlike other fats, trans-fats are neither required nor beneficial for health. Eating trans-fats increases the risk of coronary heart disease.

3. Fiber:

Fiber is a type of carbohydrate that your body doesn't 'digest' and that provides no calories. But it is important. Fiber aids in losing weight, helps to manage diabetes, relieves constipation, and helps protect against colon cancer. It may also lower your risk of heart disease.

Most of us, especially Americans, eat too little fiber. We average about 15 grams of it a day, far less than we should be eating.

Recommended amounts of fiber daily:

Men:

19-50 years old=38 grams per day of fiber
50 and older=30 grams per day

Women:

19-50 years old=25 grams per day
50 and older=21 grams per day
Pregnant=28 grams per day.

Add foods rich in fiber to your diet slowly. Beans, berries, bran, fruits, oatmeal, vegetables, and whole grains. Don't go overboard, because it takes your body a little time to adjust to the extra bulk passing through your digestive system. Always drink plenty of liquids. Fiber soaks up fluids like a sponge. This not only helps you feel fuller, longer, but helps form soft, easily passed stools.

4. Protein (prot):

Your body loses millions of cells every day. They are used up, worn out, rubbed off, and even cut off (your beard or fingernails). You need a source of protein to replace these lost cells.

Protein is found in every cell, all tissues and most substances in your body, except for urine and bile. Bones, teeth, muscles, enzymes, skin and blood, all contain protein. Active tissues, such as muscles and glands, are high in protein, while less active tissues, such as fat, have less.

Protein is made up of small building blocks called 'amino-acids'. There are 20 amino acids that the body uses to build different proteins, just like the letters in the alphabet are used to make different words. Of the 20 different amino acids found in food, 9 are known as 'essential'. These 9 must be obtained directly from the food we eat. The remaining 11, can be made in the body. When you eat many different foods, you get varying amounts of protein and varying amounts of amino acids. It is important to eat a variety of foods. Almost all foods you eat contain some protein, some more, some less. Fruits have very little protein compared to meat, cheese, beans, grains and vegetables, all of which have more.

When your body is stressed in anyway, physically or mentally, protein is lost. When it's too hot or too cold, you need extra protein. More protein is needed to replace nitrogen lost during heavy sweating. Exercise, fever, surgery, injury, infection, and broken bones, all increase the need for protein. Even emotional stress, such as losing a job or taking an exam, causes protein loss.

A quick way to estimate your daily protein needed is to divide your weight by 2.2. For example, if you weigh 150 pounds, you should be eating 68 grams of protein a day (150 divided by 2.2=68). Most people, especially Americans, eat more than their recommended level of daily protein.

Top 10 sources of protein are:

1-Beef
2-Poultry
3-Milk
4-Yeast bread
5-Cheese
6-Fish
7-Eggs
8-Fresh pork
9-Ham
10-Pasta

5. Carbohydrates (carb):

Carbohydrates include sugars, starches, and fiber found in foods. All plant foods-fruits, vegetables, beans and grains are rich in carbohydrates. Fruits have more sugar. vegetables, beans, and grains have more starch. Both have some fiber.

Sugars and starches are your body's main source of energy (or calories, or 'fuel'). When the food you eat is digested, sugar molecules move easily into the blood stream and travel to cells. There, they are burned for needed energy to keep your body working. Starch molecules are more complex. They are made up of many sugar molecules bound together. During digestion, these large starch molecules are slowly broken apart to yield smaller sugar fragments, which are sent to the cells to be converted to energy. If you eat more carbohydrates than your body needs for energy, the leftover is stored as fat.

Simple carbohydrates are foods that contain a lot of sugar. Common examples are: syrups, jelly, honey, soda, and molasses.

Complex carbohydrates are foods that contain a lot of starch. Common examples are: whole grains, cereals, beans, and vegetables. These foods are also rich in vitamins, minerals and fiber.

In the past, you were told to eat all the carbohydrates you wanted. In fact, most Americans get 50% or more of their daily calories (fuel) as carbohydrates. Today, carbohydrates are being blamed for many of our health concerns, especially overweight and obesity.

The national academy of sciences recommended dietary allowance ('RDA') for carbohydrates is 130 grams per day.
The recommendation ensures that your body has the minimum amount of carbohydrates needed to function properly. Most of us eat much more.

The food and drug administration ('FDA') recommends 300 gm of carbohydrates as the daily value ('DV')-the amount needed by the typical American consumer. This amount is probably closer to the usual carbohydrate intake of most adults.

Most professionals consider a diet with 40% or less of your daily calories should come from carbohydrates in order to be a 'low carbohydrate' diet. So if you need, say 1,800 calories per day, 40% would be about 720 carbohydrate calories per day.
To make good carbohydrate choices, choose more foods that are higher in starch and fiber and fewer foods that are higher in sugars.

"Kelly's Eating Favorites"

1-Have regular meals about every 5-6 hours with 'lite' snacks
between

2-Have more protein foods such as yogurt, tuna, beans or chicken for most meals and you will feel full longer

3-Include fruits as some of your snacks

4-If you have a craving for chocolate, try diet hot chocolate or dark chocolate with 60% or more of cacao

5-If busy work schedule, try 10 minute exercise before work, at lunch and walk in the evening. Days off, try the gym or longer periods of exercise

6-People who tend to be the best at weight loss are 'b' students who eat healthy foods 80% of the time and the other 20%.

7-South beach diet-choose wise food groups and smaller portions

8-When hungry, drink water first, eat high water foods like fruits, vegetables, cauliflower, green beans, carrots, bell peppers, vegetable low salt soups, tomato low salt soup, apples, berries and grapes

9-Walk and or exercise '30-60-90' minutes five times a week. Just 30 minutes will help prevent many chronic diseases such as diabetes and heart disease. 60 minutes of activity will help prevent weight gain. 90 minutes of activity will help prevent any weight gain and greatly improve cardiovascular condition.

10-People who 'log' what they eat, tend to lose more weight than those who don't

11-Count your fiber-should be at least 30 grams per day

12-Eat more slowly and it may help you eat less

13-Eat more onions, more garlic, more red and green vegetables

14-Check all packaged foods, especially processed foods. Compare the **'CCCFFPS'**: calories, cholesterol, carbohydrates, fat, fiber, protein and salt.

Special comments:

1. Green tea:

Drink more green tea, especially 'Long Jing, Black Dragon green tea' from Hanzhou, China. Tea is very popular in china and in fact it was invented or discovered in China over 2,000 years ago. There is some speculation that this special tea has very powerful antioxidant properties including the ability to help prevent all cancers and help prevent heart disease. The rule of thumb is that the lighter the tea is, the more healthy it may be.

2. Organic foods:

Organic foods are crops that were grown without conventional pesticides, artificial fertilizers, sewage sludge and were processed without ionizing radiation or food additives. In animals, for food, no growth hormones were used. Also, no genetic modified organisms were used. Organic foods may be more sustainable and environmentally sound

3. Fresh foods:

Fresh, 'unprocessed' organic foods such as vegetables and fruits are purchased direct from growers, farmer markets, food stands and supermarkets. Animal unprocessed meats, eggs and dairy are much less common.

Chapter Five: Secret # Three-Counter Chart

This chapter is a 'chart' listing many popular foods and meals and how much of the "7" Food Factors: Calories (cal), Proteins (prot), Fats, Cholesterol (chol), Carbohydrates (carb), Fiber (fib) and Sodium (sod, na, salt) they contain.

This "counter chart" is an excellent reference to compare foods and help decide which foods or meals may be more healthy. It's important to check all "7" categories, because, even if a food has very little cholesterol, for example, it may be loaded with fat or salt (sod).

The first few pages are not in alphabetical order, but are some of the more popular or common foods and snacks. After that list, beginning with 'apple', the list follows a more alphabetical pattern for easier review.

Calories Counter:

1. Serving size, amount (amt)-generally around 3 ounces or ½ cup or exact amount will be shown. These 'amounts' were set by national standards and may be understated. For example, beef porterhouse steak, the seven food factors that are listed compared to three ounce quantity. Most folks, especially men, will likely eat more than that. So, if a person eats nine ounces, then each 'food factor' would need to be multiplied by three.

2. Quantities or amounts: remember that:

1-Calories-amount of 'fuel' or standard of energy

2-Protein-listed in grams

3-Fat-listed in grams

4-Cholesterol-listed in milligrams

5-Carbohydrates-listed in grams

6-Fiber-listed in grams

7-Sodium (sod, na, salt)-listed in milligrams

FOOD AMT Cal Prot Fat Chol Carb Fib Sod

FOOD	AMT	Cal	Prot	Fat	Chol	Carb	Fib	Sod
Coffee mate	Tsp	10	0	0.5	0	1	0	0
Triscuits-low fat	7	120	3	3	0	21	3	160
Cheez-Its-low fat	29	130	4	4	0	20	1	360
Krispy saltines	5	60	1	1.5	0	11	1	190
Snyders-pretzels	16	120	3	0	0	25	1	200
Wheat thins-low fat	16	130	3	4	0	21	1	260
Snyders unsalted pretzels	20	110	3	0	0	25	1	75
Fiber one cereal	½ cup	60	2	1	0	25	14	105
Fat free milk	1 cup	90	8	0	5	11	0	125
Teriyaki sauce	1 tbsp	15	1	0	0	2	0	610
Ranch dressing lite-HV	2 tbsp	80	1	7	5	3	0	280
Parmesan cheese	1 tbsp	20	2	1.5	5	0	0	120
Butter	1 tbsp	100	0	11	30	0	0	95
Mayonnaise	1 tbsp	100	0	11	5	0	0	75
Mustard	1 tsp	0	0	0	0	0	0	55
BBQ sauce	2 tbsp	40	0	0	0	11	0	420
Vegetable oil	1 tbsp	120	0	14	0	0	0	0
Olive oil ex light	1 tbsp	120	0	14	0	0	0	0
Raisins	¼ cup	130	1	0	0	31	2	10
Mac & cheese ½ fat-Kraft	3 ½ oz	290	13	4.5	15	50	2	850
Zatarains New Orleans yellow rice	57 gms	190	4	0	0	43	1	920
Sloppy Joe sauce	64 gms	30	1	0	0	6	0	380
Peanut butter low fat	2 tbsp	190	8	11	0	15	2	160
Spam-turkey	2 oz	80	10	4	30	1	0	420
Baked beans	½ cup	150	7	1	0	29	7	550
Green beans can	½ cup	20	1	0	0	4	1	400
Early peas can	½ cup	60	4	0	0	12	3	380

FOOD	AMT	Cal	Prot	Fat	Chol	Carb	Fib	Sod

Food/Amt/Cal/Prot/Fat/Chol/Carb/Fib/Sod

FOOD	AMT	CAL	PROT	FAT	CHOL	CARB	FIB	Sod
Multi-grain bread	1 slice	110	5	1.5	0	19	5	180
Deli cheese-jalapeno	1 slice	80	5	6	15	2	0	320
Chicken fillets-breast	1	240	19	9	30	20	0	680
Equal artificial sweetener	1	0	0	0	0	0	0	0

Alphabetical listing begins:

FOOD	AMT	CAL	PROT	FAT	CHOL	CARB	FIB	Sod
Apple medium	1	81	0	0	0	21	2	0
Artichoke cooked	1	60	4	0	0	13	7	114
Fried rice with ckn & egg	1 meal	330	12	9	60	51	5	1270
Teriyaki chicken	¾ cup	399	30	27	92	7	0	2190
Asparagus	½ cup	22	2	0	0	4	1	10
Avocado mashed	1 cup	407	5	40	0	16	11	29
Bacon 3 strips	3	156	10	12	36	0	0	714
Bagel plain	1	190	20	5	0	18	11	310
Banana medium	1	109	1	0	0	28	3	1
Beer Bud light	12 0z	110	0	0	0	7	0	0
Beer Corona	12 0z	148	0	0	0	9	0	0
Beer Heineken	12 oz	166	0	0	0	10	0	0
Blueberries	1 cup	82	1	1	0	20	0	9
Raisin bread	1 slice	71	2	1	0	14	0	101
White bread	1 slice	67	2	1	0	12	1	135
Whole wheat	1 slice	70	3	1	0	13	2	149
Broccoli	½ cup	12	1	0	0	2	1	12
Brussels sprouts	1	8	1	0	0	2	0	4
Cabbage	½ cup	9	1	0	0	2	0	6
Cheesecake	2.8 oz	256	4	18	44	20	2	165
Pound cake	1 oz	117	2	6	66	15	0	119
Yellow cake w frosting	2.2 oz	242	2	11	35	36	1	216
Gingerbread	2.6 oz	264	3	12	24	36	2	242
Angel food cake	1.8 oz	129	3	0	0	29	1	255
Canadian bacon grilled	6 oz	257	34	12	81	2	0	2149
Caramels	2.5 oz	271	3	6	5	55	0	174
Dark chocolate	1 oz	150	1	10	0	16	0	5

FOOD	AMT	Cal	Prot	Fat	Chol	Carb	Fib	Sod
Jelly beans large	10	104	0	0	0	26	0	7
Peanut brittle	1 oz	128	2	5	4	20	0	128
Baby Ruth bar	2.1 oz	270	4	13	0	36	2	130
Butterfinger bar	2.1 oz	270	3	11	0	42	1	130
Milk choc w almonds	0.6 oz	100	2	6	5	9	0	10
Snickers	2.0 oz	240	3	11	5	32	1	80
Cantaloupe	1 cup	57	1	0	0	13	1	14
Carrots	2.5 oz	31	1	0	0	7	2	25

Food/Amt/Cal/Prot/Fat/Chol/Carb/Fib/Sod

FOOD	AMT	CAL	PROT	FAT	CHOL	CARB	FIB	
Cauliflower	2.2 oz	20	2	0	0	4	2	15
Celery	1.3 oz	6	0	0	0	1	1	35
Bran flakes cereal	¾ cup	90	4	1	0	22	0	264
Corn flakes	1 & ¼ cup	110	2	0	0	22	0	264
Oatmeal instant w water	8.2 oz	138	6	2	0	24	4	377
Shredded Mini Wheats	1 cup	107	3	1	0	24	3	3
Cheerios	1 cup	110	3	2	0	22	0	210
Grape nuts	½ cup	200	7	1	0	47	6	310
Raisin bran	1 cup	200	6	2	0	47	8	370
Champagne	4 oz	84	0	0	0	4	0	4
Cheese American	1 oz	93	6	7	18	2	0	332
Cheese cheddar	1 oz	114	7	9	30	0	0	230
Cheese low fat cheddar	1 oz	49	9	2	6	1	0	174
Cheese mozzarella	1 oz	80	6	6	22	1	0	106
Cheese provolone	1 oz	100	7	8	20	1	0	248
Cheese swiss	1 oz	107	8	8	26	1	0	74
Yogurt cheese	1 oz	80	6	7	15	0	0	60
American cheese w jalapeno	1 oz	80	6	6	20	2	1	260
Muenster cheese	1 oz	100	6	8	25	0	0	140
Beef round lean-no fat	3 oz	193	26	26	82	0	0	43
Beef brisket	3 oz	183	26	8	81	0	0	53
Beef eye round fat trimmed	3 oz	153	24	5	59	0	0	53
Beef ground ex lean broiled	3 oz	217	22	14	71	0	0	59

FOOD	AMT	Cal	Prot	Fat	Chol	Carb	Fib	Sod
Beef porterhouse lean-trim	3 oz	260	21	19	70	0	0	52
Beef rib eye	3 oz	261	21	19	70	0	0	54
Beef t-bone	3 oz	253	21	18	70	0	0	52
Beef tenderloin	3 oz	194	23	11	72	0	0	52
Beef top round braised	3 oz	184	30	6	77	0	0	38
Beef sirloin	3 oz	194	25	10	76	0	0	55
Chicken breast w skin	4.9 oz	364	35	18	119	13	0	385
Chicken drumstick fried w skin	2.6 oz	193	16	11	62	6	0	194
Chicken breast no skin	3 oz	110	25	2	70	0	0	30
Chicken breast tenders	3	250	12	15	40	15	0	480
Chicken wings spicey	4	280	18	20	90	9	0	450
Doritos toasted corn	1 0z	140	2	7	0	18	1	120
Fritos king	1 oz	150	2	9	0	16	1	180
Lays baked	1 oz	110	2	2	0	23	2	150
Cape cod golden chips	1 oz	140	2	8	0	16	0	150
Pringles	1 oz	160	2	11	0	15	1	170
Pringles sour cream	1 oz	160	2	10	0	15	1	135
Ruffles	1 oz	110	2	2	0	23	2	180
Nestle chips semi sweet	1 oz	136	1	9	0	18	0	3
Quick chocolate	1.3 oz	100	1	1	0	23	0	30
Coconut fresh	1.5 oz	159	2	15	0	7	4	9
Cod Atlantic fish cooked	3 oz	89	19	1	47	0	0	66
Espresso café latte	1 pkg	70	3	2	10	10	0	50
Collards	½ cup	6	0	0	0	1	0	4
Birds eye Chopped greens	1 cup	30	2	0	0	2	2	20
Keeblers chips deluxe	2	160	0	10	0	18	0	100
Mothers circus animals	6	140	1	6	0	20	0	100
Chips ahoy	3	160	2	8	0	21	0	105
Honey maid grahams	8	120	2	3	0	22	1	180
Fig Newtons	2	110	1	3	0	22	1	125
Oreo	3	160	1	7	0	23	1	220
Pepperridge choc chunk soft	2	280	2	10	10	44	2	130
Vanilla wafers Ralston	7	150	1	6	0	22	1	115
Ruffles fat free cheddar	1 0z	75	3	0	0	16	1	230
Ruffles light	1 oz	70	2	0	0	17	1	190
Voortman sugar cookies	2	160	1	8	0	22	0	90

FOOD	AMT	Cal	Prot	Fat	Chol	Carb	Fib	Sod
Canned corn whole dm	½ cup	90	2	1	0	18	3	360
Mexicorn	1/3 cup	60	2	0	0	14	1	250
Fresh corn	1 ear	77	3	1	0	17	0	14
Cottage cheese creamed	4 oz	117	14	5	17	3	0	457
Couscous cooked	1 cup	176	6	0	0	36	2	8
Canned crab blue	3 oz	84	17	1	76	0	0	283
Crab fresh Alaska cooked	1 leg	129	26	2	72	0	0	1436
Cheese crackers	2	10	0	0	0	2	0	20
Pepperidge goldfish	1 pkg	170	4	7	5	24	1	320
Cranberries fresh	1 cup	54	0	0	0	14	0	1
Cranberry juice cocktail	1 cup	147	0	0	0	38	0	10
Ocean spray cocktail	8 oz	140	0	0	0	34	0	35
Crayfish raw	3 oz	76	16	1	118	0	0	45
Cream cheese	3 oz	297	6	30	93	2	0	251
Cucumber fresh	½ cup	7	0	0	0	1	1	1
Dates dried whole	10	228	2	0	0	61	0	2
Bologna beef	1 oz	88	4	8	16	0	0	278
Salami hard pork	1 oz	123	6	12	0	9	0	678
Pastrami	2.5 oz	100	14	5	50	1	0	750
Pepperoni	1 oz	140	6	13	25	1	0	490
Chicken fingers banquet	Meal	740	22	43	70	67	6	1070
Teriyaki beef meal HC	9.5 oz	310	16	7	40	44	5	600
Teriyaki chicken meal HC	11 oz	270	15	6	40	37	6	600
Roast turkey breast HC	8.5 oz	220	18	5	25	28	5	600

Food/Amt/Cal/Prot/Fat/Chol/Carb/Fib/Sod

FOOD	AMT	CAL	PROT	FAT	CHOL	CARB	FIB	Sod
Roasted chicken Lean Cuisine	8 oz	190	17	4	35	22	4	690
Baked chicken Lean Cuisine	8.6 oz	240	17	5	30	33	3	550
Turkey breast Lean Cuisine	9.75 oz	270	13	2	25	49	3	590
Beef pot roast Swanson	14 oz	320	19	8	35	44	4	1200
Doughnuts glazed	2.1 oz	242	4	14	4	27	1	205
Doughnuts crème filled	3 oz	307	6	21	20	26	0	262
Duck roasted w skin	4.9 oz	472	27	40	118	0	0	83
Duck roasted no skin	4.9 oz	281	33	16	125	0	0	91
Egg fresh	1	75	6	5	213	1	0	63

FOOD	AMT	Cal	Prot	Fat	Chol	Carb	Fib	Sod
Egg white only	1	17	4	0	0	0	0	55
Egg deviled	2 halves	145	6	13	280	1	0	180
Sweet n sour La Choy	3 oz	220	6	9	15	29	2	550
Egg substitutes	1 & ½ oz	40	6	2	0	0	0	83
Egg beaters	1/2 cup	60	12	0	0	2	0	230
Egg plant	1.4 oz	11	0	0	0	2	0	1
Gatorade	8 oz	50	0	0	0	14	0	110
Snapple	11 oz	210	7	0	0	43	5	110
English muffins Thomas	1	120	4	1	0	25	1	200
English muffins Pepperidge	1	130	5	1	0	26	2	250
Metamucil fiber wafers	2	120	2	5	0	17	6	20
Breaded fish fillet frozen	2 oz	155	9	7	64	14	0	332
Fish oil cod	1 tbsp	123	0	14	78	0	0	0
Green Beans Canned	½ cup	13	1	0	0	3	1	170
Flounder cooked	3 oz	99	21	1	58	0	0	89
Flour all purpose	¼ cup	100	3	0	0	22	0	0
French toast frozen	2 oz	126	4	4	48	19	2	292
French toast take out w butter	2 slices	356	10	19	116	36	0	513
Garlic fresh chopped	1 tsp	4	0	0	0	1	0	1
Gelatin mix as prep	1 cup	80	2	0	0	19	0	9
Turkey giblets simmered	1 cup	243	39	7	606	3	0	85
Turkey gizzards simmered	1 cup	236	43	6	336	1	0	79
Goat roasted	3 oz	122	23	3	64	0	0	73
Goose w skin roasted	6.6 oz	574	47	41	172	0	0	132
Goose roasted no skin	5 oz	340	41	18	138	0	0	108
Grape juice	1 cup	155	1	0	0	38	0	7
Grapes fresh	10	36	0	0	0	9	0	1
Canned chicken w gravy	1 cup	189	5	14	5	13	0	1375

Food/Amt/Cal/Prot/Fat/Chol/Carb/Fib/Sod

FOOD	AMT	CAL	PROT	FAT	CHOL	CARB	FIB	
Grouper cooked	3 oz	100	21	1	40	0	0	45
Haddock cooked	5.3 oz	168	36	1	110	0	0	131
Halibut cooked	3 oz	119	23	2	35	0	0	59
Ham canned roasted	3 oz	116	18	4	26	0	0	965
Ham center cut country	4 oz	220	31	9	80	0	0	3045

FOOD	AMT	Cal	Prot	Fat	Chol	Carb	Fib	Sod
Ham Prosciutto	1 oz	55	8	2	20	0	0	765
Brandy Alexander	1 serv	266	1	6	20	12	0	17
Hamburger w bacon and cheese	1 double	457	28	28	110	22	0	635
Smoked sausage hill	2 oz	110	9	8	0	0	0	510
Hamburger single w b and cheese	1 large	609	32	37	112	37	0	1044
Hazel nuts	1 oz	191	4	19	0	5	0	1
Hickory nuts	1 oz	187	4	18	0	5	0	0
Herrings cooked	3 oz	172	20	10	65	0	0	98
Herrings smoked	3.5 oz	210	22	14	70	0	0	550
Honey	1 tbsp	64	0	0	0	17	0	1
Honeydew melon	1 cup	60	1	0	0	16	0	17
Carnation hot cocoa	1 pkg	70	3	0	0	15	0	140
Hot dog beef	2 oz	180	7	16	35	1	0	586
Hot dog pork	1.5 oz	144	5	13	22	1	0	504
Hot dog turkey	1.5 oz	102	6	8	48	1	0	642
Corn dog take out	1	460	17	19	79	56	0	972
Ice cream chocolate	½ cup	143	3	7	22	19	0	50
Ice cream vanilla	½ cup	132	2	7	29	16	0	53
Atkins indulge ice cream	½ cup	140	2	12	45	13	5	20
Klondike bar	1	280	3	19	20	24	0	75
Starbucks ice cream	½ cup	230	5	12	65	26	0	50
Jams most flavors	1 pkg	34	0	0	0	9	0	0
Ketchup Heinz	1 tbsp	15	0	0	0	4	0	190
Kidney beans	1 cup	207	13	1	0	38	9	889
Lamb cubed braised	3 oz	190	29	7	92	0	0	60
Lentils cooked	1 cup	231	18	1	0	40	0	4

Food/Amt/Cal/Prot/Fat/Chol/Carb/Fib/Sod

Food	Amt	Cal	Prot	Fat	Chol	Carb	Fib	Sod
Lettuce	1 leaf	3	0	0	0	0	0	2
Lettuce romaine	½ cup	4	0	0	0	1	0	2

FOOD	AMT	Cal	Prot	Fat	Chol	Carb	Fib	Sod
Lima beans canned	1 cup	191	12	0	0	36	0	809
Lemon fresh	1	22	1	0	0	12	0	3
Lime fresh	1	20	0	0	0	7	0	1
Apricot brandy	1 oz	96	0	0	0	9	0	0
Black Russian	1 serv	184	0	0	0	12	0	3
Bloody Mary	1 serv	150	1	0	0	5	1	332

Food/Amt/Cal/Prot/Fat/Chol/Carb/Fib/Sod

FOOD	AMT	CAL	PROT	FAT	CHOL	CARB	FIB	
Coffee liqueur	1 serv	175	0	0	0	24	0	4
Cognac	1 oz	67	0	0	0	0	0	0
Daiquiri	1.5 oz	187	0	0	0	15	0	7
Gin	1.5 oz	110	0	0	0	0	0	1
Grasshopper	1.5 oz	275	1	5	15	26	0	13
Hot buttered rum	1.5 oz	219	0	4	10	15	4	48
Mai tai	1.5 oz	165	0	0	0	17	0	51
Manhattan	1.5 oz	171	0	0	0	3	0	9
Margarita	1.5 oz	173	0	0	0	11	0	3
Mint julep	1 serv	136	0	0	0	17	0	3
Old fashion	1 serv	223	0	0	0	4	0	5
Pina Colada	4.5 oz	262	1	3	0	40	0	9
Gin & tonic	7.5 oz	171	0	0	0	16	0	10
Rum	1.5 oz	97	0	0	0	0	0	0
Southern comfort	1.5 oz	184	0	0	0	0	0	0
Tequila	1.5 oz	117	0	0	0	0	0	0
Vodka	1.5 oz	97	0	0	0	0	0	0
Liver pan fried	3 oz	184	23	7	410	7	0	90
Lobster cooked	1 cup	142	30	1	104	2	0	551
Macadamia nuts dry roasted	10-12	200	2	22	0	4	1	80
Mackerel canned	1 cup	296	44	12	150	0	0	720
Mackerel cooked	3 oz	223	20	15	64	0	0	71

Food/Amt/Cal/Prot/Fat/Chol/Carb/Fib/Sod

FOOD	AMT	CAL	PROT	FAT	CHOL	CARB	FIB	SOD
Mango fresh	1	135	1	1	0	35	0	4
Margarine tub corn	1 tsp	34	0	4	0	0	-	51

FOOD	AMT	Cal	Prot	Fat	Chol	Carb	Fib	Sod
Marlin raw	3 oz	110	20	3	0	0	0	0
Marshmallow	1	23	0	0	0	6	0	3
Mayonnaise	1 tbsp	99	0	11	8	0	0	78
Beef jerky	1 large	67	8	3	22	3	0	569
Condensed milk sweet	1 oz	123	3	3	13	21	0	49
Evaporated milk	½ cup	169	9	10	37	13	0	122
Milk 1 %	1 cup	102	8	3	10	12	0	123
Milk 2 %	1 cup	121	8	5	18	12	0	122

Food/Amt/Cal/Prot/Fat/Chol/Carb/Fib/Sod

Food	Amt	Cal	Prot	Fat	Chol	Carb	Fib	Sod
Buttermilk	1 cup	99	8	2	9	12	0	257
Skim milk	1 cup	86	8	0	4	12	0	125
Whole milk	1 cup	150	8	8	33	11	0	122
Milk shake chocolate	10 oz	360	10	11	37	58	0	273
Mullet cooked	1 cup	207	6	2	0	41	2	3
Molasses	1 cup	873	0	1	0	226	0	120
Mushrooms pieces	½ cup	19	1	0	0	4	0	0
Mussels cooked	3 oz	147	20	4	48	6	0	213
Mustard 1 tsp	5	0	0	0	0	0	0	63

Food/Amt/Cal/Prot/Fat/Chol/Carb/Fib/Sod

FOOD	AMT	CAL	PROT	FAT	CHOL	CARB	FIB	Sod
Navy beans canned	1 cup	296	20	1	0	54	0	1173
Nectarine	1	67	1	1	0	16	2	0
Noodles chow mein	1 cup	237	4	14	0	25	2	189
Ensure	8 oz	250	9	6	5	40	0	200
Viactiv calcium chew	1	20	0	1	0	0	0	0
Mixed nuts dry w salted peanuts	1 oz	169	5	15	0	7	0	223
Canola oil	1 tbsp	124	0	14	0	0	0	0
Corn oil	1 tbsp	120	0	14	0	0	0	0
Olive oil	1 tbsp	119	0	14	0	0	0	0
Peanut oil	1 tbsp	119	0	14	0	0	0	0
Vegetable oil	1 tbsp	120	0	14	0	0	0	0
Okra fresh	8	36	2	0	0	7	0	8
Olives green medium	4	15	0	2	0	0	0	312

FOOD	AMT	Cal	Prot	Fat	Chol	Carb	Fib	Sod
Olives ripe large	1	5	0	0	0	0	0	38
Spanish olives stuffed	5	15	0	1	0	1	0	320
Onion chopped fresh	½ cup	30	1	0	0	7	0	2
Scallions raw sliced	½ cup	16	1	0	0	4	1	8
Onion rings fried	8-9	275	4	16	14	31	0	430
Mandarin oranges	1	69	1	0	0	17	4	1
Tropicana Orange Juice	8 oz	110	2	0	0	26	0	0
Ostrich cooked	3 oz	120	22	3	74	0	0	57
Oysters canned	3 oz	58	6	2	46	3	0	95
Oysters raw	6 med	170	18	6	46	3	0	94
Oysters fried	6	368	13	18	109	40	0	677
Pancake syrup maple	1 tbsp	52	0	0	0	13	0	2
Pancakes	1-4 inch	74	2	1	0	14	0	239
Papaya fresh	1 cup	54	1	0	0	14	0	4
Parsley fresh	½ cup	11	1	0	0	2	0	17
Parsnips cooked	½ cup	63	1	0	0	31	0	17
Passion fruit	1	18	0	0	0	4	0	5
Pasta shells cooked small	1 cup	162	5	1	0	33	2	1
Spaghetti cooked	1 cup	197	7	1	0	40	2	1
Buitoni angel hair	1 & ¼ cup	230	10	3	50	43	2	20
Buitoni ravioli ckn parmesan	1 & ¼ cup	310	14	8	55	45	2	620
Chef Boyardee beef ravioli	1 cup	230	9	5	20	37	4	1120
Chef Boy. spaghetti &meat balls	8.4 oz	240	9	10	25	32	2	950
Beef macaroni HC	8.5 oz	220	12	4	20	34	5	450
Baked lasagna HC	9 oz	270	13	7	20	38	4	600
Pate chicken liver	1 tbsp	109	2	2	0	1	0	0

Food/Amt/Cal/Prot/Fat/Chol/Carb/Fib/Sod

FOOD	AMT	CAL	PROT	FAT	CHOL	CARB	FIB	Sod
Peach fresh	1	37	1	0	0	10	1	0
Peanut butter Jif low fat	2 tbsp	190	8	12	0	15	2	250
Peanut butter Jif chunky regular	2 tbsp	188	8	16	0	7	2	156
Peanuts dry roast w salt	30	170	7	14	0	6	2	230

Food/Amt/Cal/Prot/Fat/Chol/Carb/Fib/Sod

FOOD	AMT	CAL	PROT	FAT	CHOL	CARB	FIB	SOD

FOOD	AMT	Cal	Prot	Fat	Chol	Carb	Fib	Sod
Pears fresh	1	98	1	1	0	25	4	1
Peas canned	½ cup	59	4	0	0	11	0	186
Peas cooked	½ cup	67	4	0	0	13	0	2
Pecans dry roasted	1 oz	187	2	18	0	6	0	0
Pecans dry roasted w salt	20	200	3	21	0	4	3	110
Peppers canned green	½ cup	13	1	0	0	3	0	958
Old El Paso chiles	1 oz	5	0	0	0	1	1	110
Banana fresh	1-4 inch	9	1	0	0	2	1	4
Perch cooked	3 oz	99	21	1	98	0	0	67
Pickles dill	1-2.3 oz	12	0	0	0	3	0	833
Pickles gerkins	1 oz	6	0	0	0	1	0	274
Mrs Smith pie apple	1 slice	350	3	19	0	41	3	430
Mrs Smith pie chocolate cr	1 slice	340	3	18	15	43	2	380
Mrs Smith pie pecan	1 slice	560	6	27	65	75	2	450
Sara Lee pumpkin	4.6 oz	260	4	11	30	37	2	460
Mrs Smith key lime pie	1 slice	430	5	18	15	62	1	290
Pie crust baked	1/8 of 9 inch	82	1	5	0	8	0	104
Pine nuts dry	1 tbsp	51	2	5	0	1	0	0
Pineapple	1 slice	42	0	0	0	10	1	1
Pinto beans canned	1 cup	186	11	1	0	35	0	998
Pistachios dry salted	1 oz	172	4	15	0	8	0	260
Pizza home run cheese	1/6 pizza	240	8	12	20	25	1	580
Red Baron deep pepperoni	1 pizza	460	17	25	35	41	2	910
Totinos cheese	½ pizza	320	15	14	20	34	2	620
Plums fresh	1	36	1	0	0	9	0	0
Poi	½ cup	134	0	0	0	33	0	14
Popcorn microw or original gourmet	3 cups	92	3	1	0	22	5	2
Popcorn or microw butter	3 cups	168	2	13	0	15	4	388
Pop Secret jumbo movie	1 cup	40	0	3	0	4	0	55
Pop Secret fat free butter	1 cup	20	0	0	0	4	0	40
Pork blade roast lean	3 oz	229	20	16	73	0	0	57
Pork center loin chop	3 0z	172	25	7	72	0	0	53
Pork tenderloin	3 oz	139	24	4	67	0	0	48

Food/Amt/Cal/Prot/Fat/Chol/Carb/Fib/Sod

FOOD	AMT	CAL	PROT	FAT	CHOL	CARB	FIB	Sod

FOOD	AMT	Cal	Prot	Fat	Chol	Carb	Fib	Sod
Hormel pork roast au jus	5 oz	180	29	7	85	0	0	570
Banquet beef pot pie	7 oz	400	9	23	30	38	1	1000
Healthy choice ckn pot pie	9.5 oz	310	22	7	45	40	5	570
Swanson turkey pot pie	7 oz	440	12	24	18	44	2	748
Potato baked w skin	6.5 oz	220	5	0	0	51	0	16
Potato french fries frozen	10	111	2	4	0	17	2	15
Au gratin Betty Crocker	½ cup	150	3	6	5	22	1	600
Cheddar broccoli potatoes HC	10.5 oz	330	13	7	25	53	6	550
Hash browns Betty Crocker	½ cup	190	3	8	0	30	3	620
Idahoan mashed potatoes	½ cup	110	2	3	0	20	1	450
Baked potato w cheese/bacon	1	451	18	26	30	44	0	973
Take out french fries	1 large	355	5	19	0	44	0	187
Pretzels	1 oz	108	3	1	0	23	1	486
Pretzel rods	4	229	6	2	0	48	1	1029
Pretzel sticks	2 oz	229	6	2	0	48	2	1029
Royal gold fat free tiny twists	18	110	3	0	0	23	1	420
Sunsweet prunes dried	5	100	1	0	0	24	3	5
Pudding tapioca prep w milk-whole	5 oz	161	4	4	17	28	0	171
Hunts snack pudding choc	1 serv	143	2	5	1	22	0	139
Pumpkin seeds roasted	¼ cup	296	19	24	0	8	0	324
Pumpkin seeds roast w salt	¼ cup	296	19	24	0	8	0	653
Quiche lorraine pie	1/8 pie	600	13	48	285	29	0	653
Radishes red	10	7	0	0	0	2	0	11
Raisins seedless	1 tbsp	27	0	0	0	7	0	0
Raspberries	1 cup	61	1	1	0	14	0	0
Red beans hunts small	½ cup	89	6	1	0	19	6	713
Rhubarb	½ cup	13	1	0	0	3	0	2
Rice brown long cooked	1 cup	216	5	2	0	46	4	2
Rice white long instant	1 cup	162	3	0	0	35	1	5
La Choy fried rice	1 cup	236	5	1	0	53	2	1024
Uncle bens white prep	1 cup	170	4	0	0	38	0	0
Pillsbury rolls french	1	110	4	2	0	19	0	220
Hamburger rolls	1	123	4	2	0	22	0	241
Hot dog roll	1	123	4	2	0	22	0	241
Ham Whole Lean Roasted	3 oz	179	25	8	80	0	0	54
Kaiser roll	1	167	6	2	0	30	0	310

FOOD	AMT	Cal	Prot	Fat	Chol	Carb	Fib	Sod
Whole wheat roll	1	75	3	1	0	15	0	135
Orange roughy fish baked	3 oz	75	16	1	22	0	0	69

Food/Amt/Cal/Prot/Fat/Chol/Carb/Fib/Sod

FOOD	AMT	CAL	PROT	FAT	CHOL	CARB	FIB	Sod
All American salad ready pac	2.5 cups	15	1	0	0	3	1	10
Chef salad ready pac	1 pkg	350	21	25	70	9	2	1060
Spring mix salad ready pac	1 pkg	35	3	0	0	7	3	40
Salad dress blue cheese	1 tbsp	77	1	8	0	1	0	0
Salad dress French	1 tbsp	67	0	6	0	3	0	214
Salad dress Italian	1 tbsp	69	0	7	0	2	0	118
Salad dress thousand island	1 tbsp	59	0	6	0	2	0	109
Take out salad dress vine + oil	1 tbsp	72	0	8	0	0	0	0
Ranch salad dress	2 tbsp	150	0	17	10	0	0	210
Salmon cooked	3 oz	155	22	7	60	0	0	48
Bumble Bee salmon can	3.5 oz	180	20	10	0	0	0	490
Smoked salmon	3 oz	99	16	4	20	0	0	666
Take out salmon cake	3 oz	241	18	15	104	6	0	601
Pace picante salsa	2 tbsp	10	0	0	0	2	0	220
Sandwich Hot Pocket cheese pizza	4.5 oz	380	11	17	45	45	3	680
Chicken fillet sand take out	1	515	24	29	60	39	0	957

Food/Amt/Cal/Prot/Fat/Chol/Carb/Fib/Sod

FOOD	AMT	CAL	PROT	FAT	CHOL	CARB	FIB	SOD
Fish fillet sand w tartar	1	524	21	29	68	48	0	939
Ham & cheese sandwich	1	353	21	15	58	33	0	772
Roast beef sandwich	1	346	22	14	52	33	0	792
Submarine w salami/ cheese sandwich	1	456	22	19	35	51	0	1650
Tuna salad sandwich	1	584	30	28	47	55	0	1294
Sardines in oil	2	50	6	3	34	0	0	121
King Oscar sardines in olive oil	1 can	150	14	11	120	0	0	340
A-1 steak sauce	1 tbsp	20	0	0	0	5	0	190
Worcestershire sauce lea	1 tsp	5	0	0	0	1	0	65
Manwich sauce	¼ cup	62	1	1	0	13	1	802

FOOD	AMT	Cal	Prot	Fat	Chol	Carb	Fib	Sod
Pace enchilada sauce	¼ cup	36	0	0	0	6	0	290
Bearnaise sauce	1 oz	177	1	19	21	1	0	257
Sauerkraut canned	½ cup	22	1	0	0	5	0	780
Sausage bratwurst	3 oz	256	12	22	51	2	0	473
Sausage Italian	3 oz	268	17	21	65	1	0	765
Caesar Salad Ready Pac	1 ½ cup	15	1	0	0	2	1	5
Sausage kielbasa	1 oz	88	8	8	19	1	0	305
Sausage pork	½ oz	48	3	4	11	0	0	168
Vienna sausage canned	4 oz	315	12	28	59	2	0	1077
Turkey sausage brown/serve	3	120	10	8	35	2	0	370
Jones light sausage -50%	2	100	7	8	25	1	0	230

Food/Amt/Cal/Prot/Fat/Chol/Carb/Fib/Sod

FOOD	AMT	CAL	PROT	FAT	CHOL	CARB	FIB	Sod
Scallop fried take out	2 large	67	6	3	19	3	0	144
Scone orange	3 oz	260	6	6	30	47	2	400
Sherbet orange	4 oz	132	1	2	5	29	0	44
Shrimp canned	3 oz	102	20	2	147	1	0	143
Shrimp fried	3 oz	206	18	10	150	10	0	292
Snacks cheese puffs	1 oz	157	2	10	1	15	0	298
Snacks pork skins BBQ	1 oz	152	169	33	1	0	756	
Snacks trail mix	1 cup	693	21	44	0	67	0	343
Snacks bagels	1 & 1/3 cup	130	2	4	0	23	0	380
Cheetos crunchy	21	160	2	10	0	15	0	290
Chex Mix trad	2/3 cup	130	2	4	0	22	1	50
Glennys soy crisps	5	60	2	4	0	8	1	30
Utz cheese ball	50	150	2	9	0	16	0	260
Snapper cooked	3 oz	109	22	1	40	0	0	48
Soda cola	12 oz	151	0	0	0	39	0	14
Soda diet cola	12 oz	2	0	0	0	0	0	21
Sole fish cooked	3 oz	99	21	1	58	0	0	89
Atkins broccoli ched/bacon	1 serv	218	11	18	184	3	0	763
Soup beef canned	1 cup	16	3	1	0	0	0	782
Soup beef noodle	1 cup	84	5	3	5	9	0	952
Soup chicken noodle	1 cup	75	4	2	7	9	0	1107
Italian Sausage w pep and onions	1 cup	210	17	11	70	14	0	112

FOOD	AMT	Cal	Prot	Fat	Chol	Carb	Fib	Sod
Soup clam chowder New England w milk	1 cup	163	9	7	22	17	0	992
Soup consumme	1 cup	29	5	0	0	2	0	637
Soup tomato	1 cup	86	2	2	0	17	0	872
Soup chunk sirloin Campbells	1 cup	180	10	8	20	17	3	890
Soup chunk chicken noodle Campbells	1 cup	100	9	3	20	16	2	860
Soup Progresso ckn/rice/veg	1 cup	100	6	2	10	15	1	820
Soup Ramen noodle beef	1 pkg	280	6	11	0	40	3	1236
Wylers chicken bouillon cube	1	5	0	0	0	1	0	900
Sour cream	1 tbsp	26	0	3	5	1	0	6
Soy milk	1 cup	79	7	5	0	4	0	30
Soy sauce	1 tbsp	7	0	0	0	1	0	1024
Soybeans dried cooked	1 cup	298	29	15	0	17	0	1
La Choy soy sauce lite	1 tbsp	15	2	0	0	2	0	542
Soybeans roasted	½ cup	405	30	22	0	29	0	149
Spaghetti sauce trad dm	½ cup	60	2	1	0	15	3	590

Food/Amt/Cal/Prot/Fat/Chol/Carb/Fib/Sod

FOOD	AMT	CAL	PROT	FAT	CHOL	CARB	FIB	Sod
Spaghetti sauce w basil/garlic w oreg hunts	½ cup	15	0	0	0	3	0	350
Ragu chunky garden w tomato/g/o	½ cup	110	2	3	0	18	2	550
Spanish food tomales Vancamp	2	210	5	13	20	20	3	610
Banquet enchilada beef	11 oz	370	10	12	20	54	6	1330
Patio burrito w bean/cheese	5 oz	300	9	9	15	45	4	690
Patio enchilada chicken	12 oz	400	13	12	35	60	8	1470
Spaghetti sauce with meat	½ cup	60	3	1	4	14	3	720
Take out enchilada w cheese	5.7 oz	320	10	19	44	29	0	784
Nachos w cheese/beans/beef/peppers	8.9 oz	568	20	31	21	56	0	1800
Take out quesadilla	1	290	0	16	40	0	0	470
Spinach raw	2 cups	20	1	0	0	5	3	80
Sprouts Chun King bean sprouts	1 cup	11	1	0	0	1	1	17
Squash acorn	½ cup	57	1	0	0	15	2	4
Squash birds eye yellow	2/3 cup	15	0	0	0	2	1	15
Squid fried	3 oz	149	15	6	221	7	0	260
Squid (calamari) deep fried	1 serv	451	15	25	423	0	0	546
Strawberries	1 cup	45	1	1	0	10	4	2

FOOD	AMT	Cal	Prot	Fat	Chol	Carb	Fib	Sod
Stuffing w water prep	½ cup	251	5	15	0	25	0	627
Take out stuffing-bread	½ cup	195	4	8	0	26	3	534
Take out stuffing-sausage	½ cup	292	8	11	12	40	1	258
Sturgeon cooked	3 oz	115	18	4	0	0	0	0
Sugar brown packed	1 cup	828	0	0	0	214	0	86
Sugar powdered	1 tbsp	31	0	0	0	8	0	0
Sugar white	1 tbsp	45	0	0	0	12	0	0
Domino white sugar	1 tsp	15	0	0	0	4	0	0
Splenda sweetener	1 pkg	0	0	0	0	0	0	0
Sunflower seeds roasted salted	1 oz	165	5	14	0	7	0	195
Sushi take out calif roll	1 piece	28	1	1	1	4	0	37
Sushi take out salmon	4 pieces	250	11	7	20	37	5	590
Swamp cabbage cooked	½ cup	10	1	0	0	2	0	60
Sweet potatoes (yams) baked w skin	3 &1/2 oz	118	2	0	0	28	3	12
Sweet potato mashed	½ cup	172	3	0	0	40	3	21
Swordfish cooked	3 oz	132	22	4	43	0	0	98
Syrup corn light	1 tbsp	56	0	0	0	15	0	24
Syrup maple	1 tbsp	52	0	0	0	13	0	2

Food/Amt/Cal/Prot/Fat/Chol/Carb/Fib/Sod

FOOD	AMT	CAL	PROT	FAT	CHOL	CARB	FIB	Sod
Tarpon fresh	3 oz	87	17	2	0	0	0	70
Lipton orange tea	1 bag	0	0	0	0	1	0	0
Celestial seasonings tea	1 cup	0	0	0	0	0	0	0
Tofu fried	0.5 oz	35	2	3	0	1	0	2
Tomato canned paste	½ cup	110	5	1	0	25	6	86
Tomato sauce canned	½ cup	37	2	0	0	9	2	738
Tomato stewed canned	½ cup	34	1	0	0	8	0	325
Tomato Italian crushed	½ cup	45	2	0	0	9	1	390
Waffle Mix	7 inch	218	5	10	39	26	1	458
Tomato grape	20	30	1	0	0	6	1	0
Tomato juice Campbells	8 oz	51	2	1	0	10	2	683
Tortilla corn	1	56	1	1	0	12	1	40
La Mexicana flour tortilla	1	80	2	3	0	13	1	260
Trout baked	3 oz	162	23	7	63	0	0	57
Tuna canned light in oil	3 oz	169	25	7	15	0	0	301
Tuna light in water	3 oz	99	22	1	25	0	0	287

FOOD	AMT	Cal	Prot	Fat	Chol	Carb	Fib	Sod
Starkist chunk light in water	3oz	60	13	1	30	0	0	250
Tuna helper creamy pasta prep	1 cup	300	14	13	20	31	1	910
Bumble Bee ready to eat tuna salad fat free	3.5 oz	190	9	2	15	25	9	510
Take out tuna salad	1 cup	383	33	19	27	19	0	824
Turkey breast w skin roasted	4 oz	212	32	8	83	0	0	70
Turkey dark meat roasted w skin	3 oz	170	26	7	78	0	0	72
Turkey leg w skin roasted	1 leg	1134	152	54	466	0	0	420
Turkey light meat w skin roasted	4.7 oz	268	39	11	103	0	0	85
Turkey light no skin	4 oz	183	35	4	81	0	0	75
Take out turkey boneless breast w stuffing/cran/apple	5 oz	260	32	9	80	10	0	250
Turnips cooked	½ cup	33	1	0	0	7	0	17
Veal cutlet braised	3 oz	172	31	4	115	0	0	57
Veal ground broiled	3 oz	146	21	6	87	0	0	70
Veal sirloin w bone roasted	3 oz	171	21	9	87	0	0	71
Take out veal scallopini	8 oz	608	-	146	46	0	0	900
Vegetable juice cocktail	6 oz	34	1	00	0	8	0	664
Vegetables canned mix	½ cup	39	2	0	0	8	0	132
Vegetables peas & carrots canned	½ cup	48	3	0	0	11	0	332
Broccoli/cauliflower& carrots in cheese birds eye	½ cup	70	3	4	5	7	2	460
Stir fry broccoli birds eye	1 cup	30	2	0	0	5	2	30
Venison roasted	3 oz	134	26	3	95	0	0	46
Vinegar cider	1 tbsp	0	0	0	0	1	0	0
Vegetable Pole Beans Frozen	¾ cup	25	1	0	0	4	2	10
Progresso balsamic	2 tbsp	10	0	0	0	2	0	0
Waffles frozen	4 inch	88	2	3	0	14	1	262

Food/Amt/Cal/Prot/Fat/Chol/Carb/Fib/Sod

FOOD	AMT	CAL	PROT	FAT	CHOL	CARB	FIB	Sod
Walnuts dry halves	14	190	4	19	9	4	2	0
Water tap	8 oz	0	0	0	0	0	0	0
Aquafina wild berry	8 oz	40	0	0	0	11	0	10
Clearly Canadian spar-kling	8 oz	45	0	0	0	10	0	10
Very fine fruit 2 raspberry	8 oz	0	0	0	0	0	0	5
Water chestnuts sliced	½ cup	66	1	0	0	15	0	9
Watermelon	1 cup	50	1	1	0	11	1	3

FOOD	AMT	Cal	Prot	Fat	Chol	Carb	Fib	Sod
Wheat sprouted	1 cup	214	8	1	0	46	1	17
Wheat germ plain toasted	¼ cup	108	8	3	0	14	4	1
Whey cheese	1 oz	126	4	8	0	9	0	146
Whipped toppings	1 tbsp	8	0	0	2	0		04
Whipped non-dairy powdered prep	1 tbsp	8	0	0	0	1	0	3
White beans dried cooked	1 cup	249	17	1	0	45	0	11
Whitefish baked	3 oz	146	21	6	65	0	0	56
Whitefish smoked	3 oz	92	20	1	28	0	0	866
Wild rice cooked	1 cup	166	7	1	0	35	3	5
Wine beaujolais	4 oz	95	00	0	0	0	0	0
Wine bordeaux red	4 oz	95	0	0	0	0	0	0
Wine chianti	4 oz	101	0	0	0	0	0	0
Wine liebfraumilch	4 oz	86	0	0	0	0	0	0
Wine merlot	4 oz	95	0	0	0	0	0	0
Wine port	3.5 oz	156	0	0	0	11	0	4
Wine rose	3.5 oz	73	0	0	0	2	0	5
Wine sangria	1 serv	88	0	0	0	6	0	4
Wine sherry	2 oz	84	0	0	0	5	0	0
Vermouth dry	3.5 oz	105	0	0	0	1	0	0
Vermouth sweet	3.5 oz	167	0	0	0	12	0	0
White wine	3.5 oz	70	0	0	0	1	0	5
Wine cooler	1 serv	218	1	0	0	8	0	10
Gallo burgundy	4 oz	88	0	0	0	0	0	4
Gallo cabernet sauvignon	4 oz	88	0	0	0	0	0	0
Gallo chardonnay	4 oz	92	0	0	0	0	0	4
Yeast bakers compressed	1 cake	18	1	0	0	3	2	5
Yellow beans cooked	½ cup	22	1	0	0	5	0	2
Yogurt fruit lowfat	8 oz	225	9	3	10	42	0	121
Yogurt plain	8 oz	139	8	7	29	11	0	105
Yogurt low fat 'ice cream'	½ cup	130	4	3	10	24	0	105
Yogurt no fat	8 oz	127	11	3	11	31	0	149
Dannon yogurt chunky non fat peach	6 oz	160	7	0	5	33	0	100
Yogurt La Crème strawberry	4 oz	140	5	5	20	21	0	75
Yogurt light non fat cherry vanilla	8 oz	100	8	0	5	18	0	120
Yoplait yogurt fat free blueberry	6 oz	180	6	2	10	34	0	80

FOOD	AMT	Cal	Prot	Fat	Chol	Carb	Fib	Sod
Yoplait yogurt light banana cream	6 oz	90	6	0	5	16	0	95
Yogurt Dannon Smootie tropical fruit	10 oz	270	8	4	15	52	0	95

Food/Amt/Cal/Prot/Fat/Chol/Carb/Fib/Sod

FOOD	AMT	CAL	PROT	FAT	CHOL	CARB	FIB	Sod
Yogurt Haagen-Daz non fat chocolate	½ cup	140	7	0	5	28	0	45
Zucchini baby raw	1	3	0	0	0	1	0	0
Zucchini sliced cooked	½ cup	14	1	0	0	4	1	2
Zucchini canned Italian	½ cup	33	1	0	0	8	0	427

Food/Amt/Cal/Prot/Fat/Chol/Carb/Fib/Sod

RESTAURANT/FOOD	AMT	CAL	PROT	FAT	CHOL	CARB	FIB	SOD
Applebees burger w fries	1 serv	1274	55	79	263	90	7	2713
Applebees quesadillas	1 serv	684	31	46	99	40	4	2175
Arbys/bkst biscuit w saus	1	460	10	33	30	27	1	1150
Arbys homestyle fries med	5 oz	370	4	16	0	53	4	710
Au bon pair/bagel cinn	6 oz	540	12	7	0	123	4	470
Au bon scone orange	4.2 oz	370	10	13	115	56	2	310
Au bon egg on a bagel	7.1 oz	500	29	5	120	64	4	880
Baskins/yogurt choc non fat soft serve	1	190	0	1	5	39	0	125
Baskins Robbins ice cream chocolate	1	270	0	16	55	31	0	105
Ben & Jerry yogurt low fat black raspberry	½ cup	140	3	2	15	28	0	60
B & J ice cream cherry garcia	½ cup	250	4	15	70	20	1	80
Blimpe cookies choc chunk	1	200	2	10	15	26	1	210
Blimpe sandwich 6 sub blt	1	588	28	32	41	49	3	1596
Blimpe sandwich hot sub meatball	1	572	28	27	58	55	2	1145

Food/Amt/Cal/Prot/Fat/Chol/Carb/Fib/Sod

RESTAURANT/FOOD	AMT	CAL	PROT	FAT	CHOL	CARB	FIB	SOD
Bob Evans/country biscuit breakfast	1 serv	841	31	41	267	71	0	2387
Bob Evans lite sausage breakfast	1 serv	479	32	21	42	50	0	1011
Bob Evans sandwich fried chicken	1 serv	994	49	70	155	40	0	2002

FOOD	AMT	Cal	Prot	Fat	Chol	Carb	Fib	Sod
Bojangles/biscuit + c ham	1	270	9	15	20	26	1	1010
Bojangles southern ckn breast	1	261	16	16	76	12	0	702
Boston Mkt/1/2 chicken w skin	9.7 oz	590	70	33	280	4	0	1010
Boston Mkt chicken sandwich low fat no cheese	10 0z	430	34	5	65	62	4	910
Boston Mkt meat loaf + brn gravy	7 oz	390	30	22	120	19	1	1040
Boston pizza/chicken fingers w fries	1	1420	45	82	?	118	0	1630

Food/Amt/Cal/Prot/Fat/Chol/Carb/Fib/Sod

RESTAURANT/FOOD	AMT	CAL	PROT	FAT	CHOL	CARB	FIB	Sod
Boston Mkt Sirloin dinner w spaghetti	1	1581	100	87	?	90	0	98
Burger King/coke large	1	330	0	0	0	82	0	0
Burger King bkfst croissant w bacon/egg	1	360	15	22	195	25	0	950
BurgerKing double cheeseburger whopper	1	1070	57	70	185	53	4	1520
Burger King French Fries Large	1	500	6	25	0	63	5	880
Burger King chicken sandwich	1	560	25	28	60	52	3	1270
Carl Jrs/breakfast quesadilla	1	370	16	17	240	36	1	910
Carl Jrs sourdough breakfast	1	410	26	20	275	33	1	930
Carl Jrs Carls famous star	1	590	24	32	70	50	3	910
Carl Jrs double western cheeseburger	1	920	51	50	155	65	3	1770
Chick-fil-a/chicken sandwich	1	410	28	16	60	38	1	1300
Chick-fil-a" chicken-n-strips	4	250	25	11	70	12	0	570
Chick-fil-a waffle fries potato	1 sm	280	3	14	15	37	5	105
Chick-fil-a" nuggets	8	260	26	12	70	12	0	1090
Chipotle/black beans	4 oz	130	9	1	0	22	0	318
Chipotle" carnitas	4 oz	227	29	12	66	0	0	873

FOOD	AMT	Cal	Prot	Fat	Chol	Carb	Fib	Sod
Chipotle fajitas vegetables	3 oz	100	1	8	0	6	1	640
Churchs/ chicken fried steak w gravy	1 serv	470	21	28	65	36	1	1615
Churchs krispy tender strips	1	137	11	5		25	11	0
Churchs" tenders	6-8	411	34	15	74	32	1	1294
Cinnabon/cinnabon reg	1	670	0	34	0	0	0	0
Dairy queen/double cheese burger w bacon	8.9 oz	610	41	36	130	31	2	1380

Food/Amt/Cal/Prot/Fat/Chol/Carb/Fib/Sod

RESTAURANT/FOOD	AMT	CAL	PROT	FAT	CHOL	CARB	FIB	SOD
Dairy Queen/chicken breast filet sandwich	6.7 oz	430	24	20	55	37	2	760
Dairy Queen chili n cheese dog	5 oz	330	14	21	45	22	2	1090
DQ blizzard ice cream cookie choc chip	1 med	950	17	36	75	143	2	660
Dennys/All American slam	1 serv	816	45	67	828	3	1	1826
Dennys" senior omelette	1 serv	429	25	20	515	8	2	755
Dennys buffalo wings	12	856	92	54	500	1	1	5552
Dennys chicken strips	5	720	47	33	95	56	0	1666

Food/Amt/Cal/Prot/Fat/Chol/Carb/Fib/Sod

RESTAURANT/FOOD	AMT	CAL	PROT	FAT	CHOL	CARB	FIB	Sod
Dominos pizza/deep dish cheese only	2 slices	482	19	22	30	56	3	112
Dominos pepperoni feast	2 slices	534	24	25	57	56	3	1349
Dominos bread sticks	2	232	6	8	0	36	2	304
Dunkin donuts/donut	1	240	3	15	0	25	0	340
Dunkin donut maple frosted	1	210	3	9	0	30	0	260
Dunkin muffin blueberry	6 oz	490	8	17	75	78	2	610
Dunkin bagel-egg	1	350	11	2	25	72	0	610
Einstein bagel/egg bagel	1	340	11	3	35	69	2	510
Einstein ham bagel	1	450	26	6	45	74	3	1390
Einstein smoked turkey sandwich white deli	1	630	35	23	70	76	3	2180

FOOD	AMT	Cal	Prot	Fat	Chol	Carb	Fib	Sod
Einstein roll up Albuquerque turkey	1	790	31	39	85	81	5	2040
El polo loco/burrito classic chicken	1	580	17	22	108	66	6	1595
El polo quesadilla chicken	1	495	22	25	53	45	2	1008
El taquitos chicken	2	370	15	17	25	43	3	690
Hungry Howies/wings	6	180	12	14	70	0	0	760
Hungry Howies pizza large cheese	1 slice	175	10	4	11	24	1	387
Hungry How pizza lg cheese w pepperoni	1 slice	191	11	4	16	24	1	450
Hungry How sub steak cheese/mushroom	½ sub	491	27	15	47	64	2	914
Ihop/pancake buttermilk	1	110	3	3	30	17	0	450
Ihop country griddle	2 oz	120	3	4	35	19	0	440
Jack in Box/breakfast croissant sausage	1	570	19	37	240	41	1	1040
Jack in Box cheeseburger ultimate	1	990	41	66	130	59	2	1620
Jack in Box french fries large	1	580	6	28	0	77	6	960
Jack in Box sourdough chicken sandwich grilled	1	520	33	28	85	33	3	1330
KFC/biscuit	1	190	2	10	2	23	0	580

Food/Amt/Cal/Prot/Fat/Chol/Carb/Fib/Sod

RESTAURANT/FOOD	AMT	CAL	PROT	FAT	CHOL	CARB	FIB	SOD
KFC/extra crispy breast	1	490	34	28	135	19	0	1230
KFC original breast recipe	1	380	40	19	145	11	0	1150
KFC crispy strips	3	400	29	24	75	17	0	1250
Krispy Kreme/glazed original	1	200	2	12	5	22	0	95
Krispy Kreme glazed crème filled	1	340	3	20	5	39	0	140

Food/Amt/Cal/Prot/Fat/Chol/Carb/Fib/Sod

RESTAURANT/FOOD	AMT	CAL	PROT	FAT	CHOL	CARB	FIB	Sod

FOOD	AMT	Cal	Prot	Fat	Chol	Carb	Fib	Sod
Krystal biscuit bacon/egg/cheese	1	390	11	23	40	33	0	1090
Krystal chicken bites	1 sm	310	17	19	55	16	1	790
Little Caesars/crazy bread	1	90	3	3	0	15	0	140
Little Caesars 18" round cheese pizza	1/14	230	12	7	15	30	1	350
Little Caesars 14" meatsa	1/10	280	15	13	30	20	2	630
Manhatten bagel/plain	1	260	10	0	0	52	2	560
Manhatten egg bagel	1	270	10	2	0	53	2	710
McDonalds/bagel steak egg/cheese	8.5 oz	640	31	31	265	57	2	1540
McDonalds big breakfast	9.4 oz	710	24	48	455	45	3	1430
McDonalds biscuit sausage w egg	5.7 oz	490	16	33	245	31	1	1010
McDonalds mcmuffin egg	4.9 oz	300	18	12	235	29	2	840
McDonalds double cheeseburger	6.1 oz	480	25	27	85	37	2	1220
McDonalds chicken mc-nuggets	6	310	15	20	50	18	2	680
McDonalds french fries large	6.2 oz	540	8	26	0	68	6	350
McDonalds quarter pounder w cheese	7 oz	530	28	30	95	38	2	1250
Miami sub/cheese burger deluxe	1	859	34	65	47	32	1	736
Miami chicken philly classic	1	551	30	27	92	47	2	1033
Miami 6 sub-meatball	1	491	28	22	76	49	4	1319
Miami 6 sub-tuna	1	468	34	18	67	44	2	1068
PF Chang's/chicken w black bean sauce	1	426	63	11	0	19	0	?
PF vegetables chow fun	1	677	16	18	0	112	0	?
Panera bread/cream cheese bagel	1	190	3	18	55	2	0	210
Panera sierra turkey	1	950	40	55	40	71	4	2380
Panera smoked turkey breast sandwich	1	590	34	16	10	73	5	2320

FOOD	AMT	Cal	Prot	Fat	Chol	Carb	Fib	Sod
Panera tuna salad on Artisian multigrain sandwich	1	830	32	41	65	78	5	1790
Papa Johns/bread sticks	1	140	4	2	0	26	1	260
Papa Johns pizza orig all meats	1/8	405	18	20	41	39	2	1114
Papa Johns pizza orig sausage	1/8	336	14	14	28	38	2	894
Pizza Hut Hot wings	2	110	11	6	70	1	0	450
Papa johns/pizza thin cheese	1/8	238	10	13	17	23	1	490
Pizza hut/bread sticks	1	150	4	6	0	20	0	220

Food/Amt/Cal/Prot/Fat/Chol/Carb/Fib/Sod

RESTAURANT/FOOD	AMT	CAL	PROT	FAT	CHOL	CARB	FIB	Sod
Pizza Hut pizza fit diced chicken	1 slice	170	10	5	15	23	2	460
Pizza Hut pizza hand toss chicken	1 slice	240	12	8	25	30	2	520
Pizza Hut pizza pepperoni	1 slice	250	12	9	25	29	2	570
Pizza Hut pan chicken supreme	1 slice	280	13	12	25	30	2	530
Pizza Hut thin n crispy meat lovers	1 slice	270	13	14	35	21	2	740
Quiznos/sub turkey lite	1 sm	334	24	6	19	52	3	1909
Quiznos sub tuscan chicken salad	1 sm	326	21	6	35	45	4	1271
Red Lobster/light grilled chicken	1	527	?	14	?	38	0	?
Red Lobster jumbo shrimp dinner/lite	1	243	?	?	?	?	0	?
Ruby Tuesday/cajun chicken salad w ranch	1	636	?	46	?	16	0	?
Ruby Tues pepperoni sirloin w mushrooms	1	947	?	57	?	19	0	?
Sbarro/cheese pizza	1	450	?	14	?	?	?	990
Sbarro spaghetti w sauce	18 oz	630	?	18	?	?	?	1260
Schlotzskys/lite chicken sandwich breast	15 oz	540	?	10	?	?	?	2370
Schlotzskys sandwich orig turkey	17 oz	1020	?	51	?	?	?	3740

FOOD	AMT	Cal	Prot	Fat	Chol	Carb	Fib	Sod
Smoothie King/activator strawberry	20 oz	559	20	1	2	123	5	260
Smoothie King low fat celestial cherry hi	20 oz	285	1	0	0	69	4	22
Smoothie King pina co-lada island	20 oz	550	16	11	5	102	6	300
Wendys/big bacon classic	9.9 oz	580	34	30	100	46	3	1460
Wendys chicken breast sand	7.3 oz	430	27	16	56	46	2	750
Wendys french fries	6.7 oz	570	8	27	0	73	7	180
Wendys baked potato w bacon/ cheese stuffed hot	12.6 oz	530	16	18	25	78	7	820
Wendys jr cheeseburger deluxe	6.3 oz	360	18	16	50	36	2	860
Wendys chicken nuggets	5	230	11	16	30	11	0	470
Whataburger/biscuit w bacon, egg, cheese	1	476	17	29	252	35	0	875
Whataburger french fries large	1	514	9	26	0	66	5	413
Whataburger chicken sandwich	1	857	51	48	150	53	3	1297

Chapter Six: Secret # Four-Review of Antioxidants

Special note!

In Chapter Eight: Secret # Six"DMVS"-Dietary Minerals, Vitamins and Supplements are explained in great detail. In this chapter, Chapter Six, Secret # Four-Review of Antioxidants, only those vitamins that are considered 'antioxidant' are discussed and only their antioxidant properties. Keep in mind that many vitamins, dietary minerals and supplements have antioxidant properties, but many do not.

Also, there will be some duplication of information, because 'DMVS' are extremely important whether or not they may be an antioxidant. For example, Vitamin B-3 (Niacin) is an important vitamin because it plays an essential role in energy metabolism, but it is not considered an antioxidant. On the other hand, Calcium, a non organic chemical element, is essential in human life especially with living cells and bone formation, but it is not a vitamin and it is not an antioxidant. But it is a critical element without which human life could not exist. Vitamin C, ascorbic acid is both a powerful vitamin and an even more powerful antioxidant.

Review of Antioxidants:

Antioxidants are chemicals that reduce the rate of oxidation and there by protect human cells from damage caused by unstable molecules known as 'free radicals'. Free radical damage may lead to cancer and heart disease. Antioxidants interact with and help stabilize free radicals. They help prevent the consumption of oxygen (O-2). Reactive O-2 species such as hydrogen peroxide, super oxide anion, and free radicals such as a hydroxyl radical are very unstable, highly reactive and can damage cells by chemical chain reaction, such as lipid peroxidation, or formation of DNA adducts that could cause cancer, cell mutations or cell death. All cells contain antioxidants that serve to reduce or prevent this damage.

Antioxidants can either stop cell damage and even 'reverse it'.

Antioxidant Uses:

1-Reduce cell damage and aging

2-Reduce risk of cancer

3-Reduce risk of heart disease and strokes

4-Reduce risk of cirrhosis of liver from alcohol ingestion

5-Helps maintain a healthy brain well into old age

6-Helps prevent illness and disease

7-Improve skin health, especially sun damage

8-Helps reduce skin wrinkles

9-Helps reduce the risk of age-related macular degeneration, the leading cause of blindness among the elderly. Vitamin C, Vitamin E, Beta-carotene and zinc were found, in one study, to ward off macular degeneration, in which abnormal blood cells grow in the eye and leak blood and fluid that damage the center of the retina and blur vision

10-Helps keep the immune system in good shape

11-Helps prevent age-related neuro-degeneration (decline of the brain and nervous system)

12-Helps prevent DNA damage and therefore helps prevent cancer

13-Helps lower cholesterol and blood pressure

Foods and Drinks High In Antioxidants:

Nearly every study celebrates the use of antioxidants for better health and longer quality living. However, which antioxidants are the best or become favored, may change monthly. Here's a list of some of the best and some comments about them:

Antioxidants Recommended by The National Cancer Institute:

Antioxidants are abundant in fruits and vegetables, as well as other foods including nuts, grains, some meats, poultry and fish.

1-Beta-carotene-(antioxidant) . A form of Vitamin A, that is converted to Vitamin A as needed. It is stored in the liver. Excess Vitamin A can be harmful, but carotene is non-toxic. It is a powerful antioxidant and is useful in curbing excess damage from free radicals. Sources include from yellow, orange and green leafy fruits and vegetables, carrots, spinach, lettuce, tomatoes, sweet potatoes, broccoli, cantaloupe, oranges, and winter squash and orange bell peppers.

2-Lutein-strong antioxidant associated with healthy eyes and is abundant in green, leafy vegetables such as collard greens, spinach, and kale

3-Lucopene-potent antioxidant found in tomatoes, watermelon, guara, papaya, apricots, pink grapefruit

4-Selenium-is not an antioxidant nutrient, but is a component of antioxidant enzymes. Sources include rice, wheat, meats, breads, and brazil nuts.

5-Vitamin A- there are 3 forms, a-1 (retinol), a-2 (3,4 didehydroretinol), and a-3 (hydroxy retinol). Sources include liver, sweet potatoes, carrots, milk, egg yolks, and mozzarella cheese

6-Vitamin C-(ascorbic acid)-one of the most powerful of all antioxidants. Sources include many fruits, vegetables, cereals, beef, poultry, and fish

7-Vitamin E-(alpha-tocopherol)-antioxidant found in almonds, oils, such as wheat germ, safflower, corn and soybean oils and in mangos, nuts and broccoli.

Antioxidants Help Preserve Health

Research suggests that antioxidant-rich foods reduce damage to cells and biochemicals from free radicals. The antioxidant chemicals reduce and may even reverse oxidative cell and biochemical damage. They help reduce cardiovascular disease by reducing the 'LDL' (lousy cholesterol) oxidants. They help reduce atherosclerosis, arteriosclerosis, and cardiovascular disease by lessening inflammation and plaque formation and other complex bio processes. But there are still many questions and answers still needed. There are literally hundreds of antioxidants and just exactly how each works independently or in combination or in excess quantities is still not completely understood.

Some antioxidants can be powerful agents against tumors but some may also, interfere with certain cancer treatments. Some studies suggest that high doses (especially by adding some supplements in addition to an already healthy diet) may cause an increase in the formation of free radicals.

However, if one looks back at some of the Nobel winning scientists, such as Linus Pauling, for example, he not only promoted many vitamin supplement additions, but he even recommended mega doses, especially with Vitamin C. Such doses may have been as high as 6,000-18,000 mg per day of C. Dr Pauling was a pioneer, along with several others in biochemical research, especially with Vitamins. He lived to be nearly a 100. From a research point of view, longevity is increased with a better healthy lifestyle by taking antioxidants (and vitamins) to live longer.

What About Exercise and Antioxidants?

By exercising, oxygen consumption can temporarily increase by a factor of 10. This may lead to a large increase in production of oxygen free radicals, resulting in increased cell damage contributing to muscle fatigue during and after exercise. The body uses antioxidants to reduce this potential damage. Increased free radicals occur especially during 24 hour period after exercise. The immune system response to this damage done by exercise, peaks, 2-7 days after the exercise.

Although it may seem, that this may be a good time to add excessive antioxidants, it may be that only certain antioxidant additions may be called for. The body and immune system quickly reacts naturally by providing its own antioxidants and supplementing 'extra' may not be called for. However, the long term benefits of regular exercise, can be proven to be extremely beneficial to better health and more resistance to disease. Some studies suggest that extra E, C, Beta-carotene, and Selenium may be beneficial in the permanent lowering of free radicals.

In one study, Mayo Clinic Newsletter report said, **"The best way to reduce and even possibly reverse aging is exercise".**

Antioxidants for nutrition

Antioxidants from diet are necessary for healthful lives in humans and several other mammals. Recently, there has been a tremendous amount of evidence suggesting that supplementation along with the diet or eating with various antioxidants can improve health and extend life. Some of the most popular antioxidant dietary supplements are Resveratrol (grape skins, especially from Cabernet type wines), combinations like 'ACES' (Beta-carotene[provitamin a], Vitamin C, Vitamin E, and Selenium) or specialty herbs known to contain antioxidants, such as green tea and jiaogulan (also known as southern ginseng or xiancao herb, and as the 'immortality herb').

Vitamins: (for more Vitamin details, see Chapter Eight, Dietary Minerals, Vitamins and Supplements)

1-Vitamin A (retinol)-

-Synthesized by the body from Beta carotene
-Helps protect body from solar radiation
-Important to healthy eyes

-Sources: carrots, squash, broccoli, sweet potatoes, tomatoes, kale, collards, cantaloupe, peaches, and apricots

2-Vitamin C (ascorbic acid)-

-Perhaps the most powerful human antioxidant, fulfills several roles in living systems: improves blood vessel and cardiovascular activity, enhances healthy hormone actions, promotes immune system, enhances nitrous oxide functions, rebuilds powerful antioxidant glutathione, promotes iron balance, reduces accumulations of toxins, improves intestinal transit time, protects DNA from damage, enhances natural anti-cancer functions, rebuilds Vitamin E and Selenium, maintains integrity of cartilage, bones, teeth, increase cellular resistance to many common viral infections and overall increase in energy and improved sense of well being.

-Sources: citrus fruits, oranges, sweet limes, green peppers, broccoli, green leafy vegetables, strawberries, blueberries, raw cabbage, and tomatoes.

3-Vitamin E (tocotrienol and tocopherol)

-E is another significantly powerful antioxidant said to help reduce cardiovascular disease, reduce cataracts, enhance the immune system, reduce cancer risk, reduce macular degeneration, reduce risk of dementia, and helps fight infection

Vitamin Co-Factors and Minerals

1-Coenzyme Q-10 (coq10) is an antioxidant but not considered a vitamin in humans. It can be manufactured by the body, but quantities decrease with age

-Uses-improve gum health and helps protect brain against Parkinson disease

2-Selenium-a trace mineral and antioxidant

-Uses-helps reduce the occurrence of male prostate cancer

-Sources-fish, shellfish, red meat, grains, eggs, sunflower seeds, chicken, turkey, garlic, brazil nuts and vegetables

3-Zinc-trace mineral and antioxidant

-Uses-essential component of many enzymes involved in digestion, metabolism, and reproduction. It also protects against premature aging of skin and muscles. In larger doses, it may help speed up healing process after injury and is used in throat lozenges or tablets to help remedy the common cold.

-Sources-oysters, some animal proteins, beans, nuts, whole grains, pumpkin seeds, and sunflower seeds

4-Manganese-plays a role in skeletal development and maintenance

Antioxidant hormones

1-Melatonin-is a natural hormone, occurs in every organism and has many biological roles. It is also a powerful antioxidant

-Uses-helps prevent DNA damage by some carcinogens and thereby stopping mechanisms of some cancers. May also reduce damage caused by Parkinson disease. May also help prevent cardiac arrhythmia and increase longevity. It may also help fight disease. Also used most commonly to help alleviate sleep disorders. Also used as a preventative treatment for migraines and cluster headaches.

-Sources-naturally synthesized by the pineal gland, retina and gastrointestinal tract

Antioxidants-Carotenoid Terpenoids

1-Lycopene-one of the most potent cartenoid antioxidants

-Uses-helps eliminate singlet oxygen, prevent skin aging, reduces risk of cardiovascular disease, cancer (especially prostate cancer), diabetes, osteoporosis, male infertility, also reduces risk of esophageal, colorectal and oral cancer

-Source-ripe red tomatoes

2-Lutein-

-Uses-health benefits to the eye, especially the retina

-Source-spinach and red peppers

3-Alpha-carotene-body converts this and 'beta' to Vitamin A

-Uses-maintenance of healthy skin, bones, good vision and a stronger immune system

-Source-carrots, sweet potatoes, squash, broccoli, kale, brussels sprout, spinach, mangos, cantaloupe

4-Beta-carotene-converts to Vitamin A as needed

-Uses-high powered antioxidant and is used in curbing excess damage from free radicals

-Source-butternut squash, carrots, orange bell peppers, sweet potatoes, pumpkins

5-Zeaxanthin-

-Uses-filters out harmful light rays and supports the retinal and muscular health of the eye

-Source-yellow corn

6-Astaxanthin-

-Uses-prevents night blindness, tired eyes, promotes gastric health, increases physical endurance, muscle recovery and anti-wrinkle

-Source-red algae, salmon

7-Canthaxantin-

-Uses-antioxidant

-Source-salmon

Non-Cartenoid Terpenoids

1-Eugenol-

-Uses-highest oxygen radical absorbance capacity of all food born substances. Used in dentistry, natural analgesic, in medicines to remedy bronchitis, common cold, cough, fever, sore throat and infections

-Source-clove oil

2-Saponins and Limonoids-

-Uses-reduce cholesterol, veterinary foot and mouth disease, anti-cancer properties, anti-inflammatory, weight loss and blood cleanser

-Source-many plant skins, licorice, olives

Flavanoid Polyphenolics (Bioflanonoids)

1. Flavonols:

1-Resveratrol-

-Uses-anti-cancer, anti-viral, anti-aging, anti-inflammatory, and prolongs life

-Source-skins of dark colored grapes and concentrated in red wine, especially cabernets

2-Pterostilbene-analogue of Resveratrol

-Uses-reduces risk of cardiovascular disease and cancer

-Source-found in Vaccinium berries

3-Kaempferol-

-Uses-helps prevent oxidative damage to human cells, lipids, and DNA. Helps prevent arteriosclerosis and blood platelet formation

-Source-apples, onions, leeks, citrus fruits, St Johns Wort

4-Myricetin-

-Uses-anti-inflammatory, antibacterial, anti-viral, anti-tumor, anti-amyloid fibril formation, and anti-alzheimers disease

-Source-walnuts

5-Isorhamnetin-

-Uses-anti-tumor, reduces free radicals and oxidative stress and diminishes lipid peroxidation

-Source-apples, onions

6-Proanthocyanidins (condensed tannins)-

-Uses-helps to reduce excess cholesterol, reduces risk of heart disease, brain loss and improves immune deficiencies

-Source-pine bark, grape seed extract, and red wine extract

2. Flavones

1-Quercetin (related to Rutin, or Rutoside)-

-Uses-helps prevent cancer, heart disease, cataracts, allergies, inflammation, respiratory diseases such as asthma and bronchitis. In some countries, it is used as a tea to induce a miscarriage

-Source-apples, black and green teas, onions, red wine, red grapes, citrus fruits, broccoli, leafy green vegetables, cranberry, raspberry, honey, and buckwheat

2-Luteolin-

-Uses-helps prevent inflammation, promotes carbohydrate metabolism, improves immune system and helps prevent cancer

-Source-parsley, thyme, peppermint, basil, celery and artichoke

3-Apigenin-

-Uses-anti-inflammatory, anti-tumor, helps reduce formation of uric acid (helps prevent gout)

-Source-parsley, thyme, peppermint, herbs, such as chamomile, lemon balm, and perilla

4-Tangeritin-

-Uses-anti-tumor, protects nerve cells

-Source-tangerines, and other citrus peels

3. Flavanones

1-Hesperetin (metabolizes to Hesperidin)-

-Uses-anti-inflammatory, anti-allergy, reduces lipid accumulation, helps protect vessels, anti-cancer and lowers cholesterol

-Source-lemons, oranges

2-Naringenin (metabolizes to Naringin)-

-Uses-enhances eyesight, reduces free radicals, anti-inflammatory, promotes carbohydrate metabolism, helps repair DNA, anti-cancer, helps reduce hypertension, helps build immune system

-Source-citrus fruits

3-Eriodictyol-

-Uses-helps prevent acute pulmonary insufficiency, helps reduce tinnitus (ringing of the ears), anti-inflammatory

-Source-herbs, citrus fruits, Resveratrol, nuts, wine, and grapes

4. Flavan-3-ols (Anthocyanidins)

1-Catechin-

-Uses-helps reduce atherosclerotic plaque, anti-cancer

-Source-chocolate, fruits, wine, berries

2-Gallocatechin-

-Uses-helps reduce atherosclerotic plaque, anti-cancer

-Source-chocolate, fruits, wine

3-Epicatechin (and its Gallate forms)-

-Uses-helps reduce atherosclerotic plaque, and anti-cancer

-Source-chocolate, fruits, wine

4-Epigallocatechin (and its Gallate forms)-

-Uses-helps reduce atherosclerotic plaque, anti-cancer

-Source-chocolate, fruits, wine

5-Theoflavin (and its Gallate forms)-

-Uses-helps control bleeding, helps heal wounds, helps regulate body temperature, helps regulate blood sugar, promotes digestion, helps heart, prevents fatigue, improves urinary and brain function, helps reduce risk of cancer

-Source-tea leaves, berries, beer, wine, chocolate, walnuts, peanuts, olive oil, fruits and vegetables

5. **Isoflaone Phytoestrogens (are antioxidants and they help protect and maintain the skeletal system)**

1-Genistein-

-Uses-anti-cancer, helps reduce risk of cancer of the breast, colon and prostate, may increase the risk of leukemia

-Source-soybeans

2-Daidzein-

-Uses-anti-cancer, decreases breast, colon and prostate cancer, but does not increase the risk of leukemia

-Source-soybeans

3-Glycitein-

-Uses-anti-cancer, decrease breast, colon and prostate cancer, but does not increase the risk of leukemia

-Source-soybeans

6. **Anthocyans**

1-Cyanidin-

-Uses-protects plants from 'ultraviolet' damage, reduces free radical damage, protects cells from oxidative change, decreases the risk of heart and cancer disease, may also help prevent obesity, diabetes, and is anti-inflammatory

-Source-berries, apples, plums

2-Delphinidin-

-Uses-food additives for color, may help prevent diabetes, cancer as well as many other antioxidant properties

-Source-cabernet wines, grapes, cranberries, fruits, flowers, stems, and roots

3-Malvidin-

-Uses-also used as food color additives, may help prevent diabetes, cancer, many other antioxidant properties

-Source-red wines, especially cabernets, grapes, cranberries, fruits, flowers, stems and roots

4-Pelargonidin-

-Uses-food color additives, may help prevent cancer, diabetes, and other antioxidant properties

-Source-red wines, red, purple, and blue fruits and vegetables

5-Peonidin-

-Uses-food color additives, may help prevent cancer, diabetes, and other antioxidant properties

-Source-red wines, red, purple, and blue fruits and vegetables

6-Petunidin-

-Uses-food color additives, may help prevent cancer, diabetes, and other antioxidant properties

-Source-red wines, red, purple, and blue fruits and vegetables

7. Phenolic Acids and their Esters

1-Ellagic acid-

-Uses-anti-cancer, helps reduce risk of heart disease, birth defects, liver problems, promotes wound healing

-Source-pomegranates, berries, red wine tannins (in their ester form), pecans, walnuts, raspberries, strawberries

2-Gallic acid-

-Uses-used to make mescaline, astringent, helps prevent night sweats and polyuria

-Source-gallnuts, sumac, witch hazel, tea leaves, oak bark and other plants

3-Salicylic acid-

-Uses-in the past, it was used as a source of making aspirin, now used to make cosmetic preps, especially to treat acne, psoriasis, callouses, corns, warts, keratosis, dandruff, used in preparation of Pepto-Bismol, also used for nausea, vomiting, and diarrhea, heartburn and gas

-Source-most vegetables, fruits, and herbs, but mostly in bark of willow trees

4-Rosmarinic acid-

-Uses-inhibits seasonal allergic rhinoconjuctivitis, type one allergy, anti-inflammatory, anti-carcinogenic, increases the tolerance to pollen

-Source-rosemary, oregano, lemon balm, sage, and marjoram

5-Cinnamic acid (and derivatives)-

-Uses-in some pharmaceuticals, perfumes, used in flavors, anti-bacterial, antifungal, anti-parasite

-Source-seeds of plants, as in brown rice, whole wheat, oats, coffee, apple, artichoke, peanuts, orange and pineapple

6-Chlorogenic acid-

-Uses-anti-tumor, anti cardiovascular disease, antibacterial and used in cosmetics

-Source-coffee, blueberries and tomatoes

7-Chicoric acid-

-Uses-increases resistance to disease, and infections, help cure snake bites, and possibly aids in its treatment

-Source-herb Echinacea Purpurea

8-Gallotannins-

-Uses-anti-inflammatory, anti-cancer, anti-viral

-Source-food grains and fruits

9-Ellagitannins-

-Uses-promotes proper cell division, helps shield against environmental toxins, increases wound healing

-Source-raspberries, blackberries

9. Other Non-Flanonoid Phenolics

1-Curcumin-

-Uses-increases wound healing, anti-inflammatory, increases heart and circulation health, anti-tumor, free radical scavenger, helps reduce risk of and state of alzheimers

-Source-rhizomes of the ginger family, turmeric (curry powder) spice

2-Anthoxanthius-

-Uses-exerts many antioxidant properties

-Source-blossoms, fruits, leaves of some plants and berries

3-Beta Cyanins-

-Uses-food dye (causes red urine and stools), remedy for constipation, and inflammation of the urinary system

-Source-beets, some flowers, and some fungi

4-Silymarin-

-Uses-treatment and prevention of liver diseases, helps prevent some cancers, of skin and prostate

-Source-milk thistle

5-Citric acid-

-Uses-natural preservative in foods and soft drinks, occurs in metabolism of almost all living things

-Source-citrus fruits and vegetables, mostly in lemon and limes

6-Lignan-

-Uses-anti-cancer, anti-tumor, viral hepatitis and liver protection

-Source-oats, flax seeds, pumpkins seeds, sesame seeds, rye, soybeans, broccoli, beans, and some berries

10. Antinutrients

1-Oxalic acid-

-Uses-strong antioxidant that readily binds to needed dietary minerals, rendering them unabsorbable in the 'GI' tract, also uses in bleaches

-Source-many plants, especially sorrel, buckwheat, rhubarb, black pepper, parsley, poppy seed, spinach, beets, cocoa, chocolate, tea plants and most nuts

2-Phytic acid (Inositol)-

-Uses-helps prevent colon cancer and other cancers, also used as a food additive

-Source-bran, seeds, nuts and grains

11. Bilirubin

-Uses-helps prevent oxidative damage from free radicals, and may help prevent cardiovascular disease

-Source-breakdown product of blood

12. Uric acid

-Uses-excess can lead to gout arthritis, deficiency associated with multiple sclerosis, antioxidant properties

-Source-occurs naturally in human body, externally from animal organs, sweetbreads, anchovies, sardines, liver, kidneys, scallops, mackerel, game meats, pork, poultry and some vegetables and bran

13. R-alpha-Lipoic Acid

-Uses-treatment of macular degeneration, increases liver health, increases memory, decreases risk of diabetes, decreases risk of alzheimer and parkinson disease, helps in several poison aids, and used as a topical anti-aging preps

-Source-spinach, broccoli, beef, yeast, and some organ meats

14. N-Acetylcysteine (RX as Mucomyst, Mucosil, Parvolex, and Hexal Ag)

-Uses-helps with emphysema, bronchitis, tuberculosis, pneumonia, helps reduce cocaine craving, used as an aid to influenza

-Source-pharmaceutical preparation and is a derivative of amino acid, l-cysteine and a precursor in formation of antioxidant, glutathione, also from whey protein

Beverages and Foods Highest in Antioxidant Properties: (per Wikipedia)

1. Undutched cocoa powder
2. Dark, semisweet chocolate: best 85% of cocoa solids
3. White tea
4. Green Rooibos (tea)
5. Green tea
6. Red Rooibos (tea)
7. Oolong tea
8. Black tea
9. Blueberries, wild-high in anthocyanins, chlorogenic acid, ellagic acid, catechins, and resveratrol
10. Blackberry and raspberry
11. Cranberry
12. Cherry (sour)
13. Dried plum prune
14. Crowberry
15. Kiwi
16. Pomegranate-high in tannins
17. Papaya-high in vitamin e and beta-carotene
18. Grapes (dark)-high in polyphenol resveratrol, tannins
19. Citrus fruits-oranges, grapefruits, pulp, best source of antioxidants

20. Dark leafy green vegetables such as broccoli (high in lutein, sulforaphane, indoles, carotenoids, beta-carotene, and zeaxanthin), brussels sprouts (high in glucosinates), and cabbage, red and green, and kale
21. Artichokes
22. Asparagus
23. Avocado
24. Beans
25. Beets
26. Carrots
27. Red peppers
28. Russet potatoes
29. Spinach
30. Tomatoes
31. Olive oil, especially, extra virgin (some studies suggest, that it reduces blood pressure, reduces LDL and fights off cancer)

Fruits and vegetables

Generally, the deeper and richer the color, denotes higher quantities of antioxidants. And many are high in fiber, minerals and vitamins. Some of the most common fruits and vegetables such as apples, bananas, iceberg lettuce and potatoes may contain very little antioxidants. It is the same with many fruit juices and drinks. Most antioxidants are in the skins and pulps.

Teas are different in that the darker varieties have less antioxidants

32. Nuts-are high in polyphenols and are highly beneficial because of their unsaturated fatty acids. They help reduce the risk of heart disease. Walnuts, pecans, hazel nuts and almonds are considered the most powerful antioxidant nuts.
33. Herbs and spices-even in small amounts, some spices are extremely high in antioxidants, especially, allspice, cinnamon, cloves, ginger, oregano, peppermint, rosemary, sage, thyme, lemon balm, and teas (white and green)

34. Seeds and grains-especially sunflower seeds and oats
35. Plants-especially cacao (cocao) and chocolate-the darker and more bitter, the higher concentrations of polyphenols

Top 20 Foods with Highest Antioxidants per USDA:

1. Small red beans
2. Wild blueberries
3. Red kidney beans
4. Pinto beans
5. Cultivated blueberries
6. Cranberries
7. Artichokes
8. Blackberries
9. Prunes
10. Raspberries
11. Strawberries
12. Red delicious and granny smith apples
13. Pecans
14. Sweet cherries
15. Black plums
16. Russet potatoes
17. Black beans
18. Plums
19. Gala apples
20. Walnuts

Foods That Score Well In Oxygen Radical Absorbance Capacity:

1. Beets
2. Brussels sprouts
3. Kale

4. Spinach
5. Many of the same berries that have total antioxidant capacity

Remember: eat good balanced meals with lots of fruits, vegetables, nuts and grains. Back off from processed foods that may be loaded with sodium, excess cholesterol and fat and also low in fiber. Eat more fresh food that is lower in fat, lower in cholesterol and lower in sodium. All these good fruits, vegetables, nuts, drinks should provide plenty of antioxidant protection without taking too many extra supplements. However, Vitamin C supplement is still strongly recommended along with complete Multi-Vitamins, Minerals, Omega-3's and some Vitamin E.

Kelly's Favorite Antioxidants:

1. Coffee in the morning, green tea (be sure to chew some of the leaves, it's ok and helps promote antioxidant action) in the afternoon, later, around dinner time, 2 glasses of red wine, cabernet, one just before dinner and one during dinner.

2. Breakfast-7 days a week:

1-Fiber One cereal (or other high fiber cereal)
2-add ½ tbsp of blueberries, fresh or dried
3-add ½ tbsp of cranberries, dried
4-add ½ tbsp of unsalted almonds
5-add ½ tbsp of unsalted walnut halves
6-add 6-8 ounces of skim (fat free) milk

3. Shortly after finishing breakfast, take the following antioxidants and supplements:
1-Vitamin C 1,000-1,500 mg extended release daily
2-Vitamin E 400 mg

3-Omega 3 fish oil 1000 mg enteric coated, 1-3 daily depending on your cholesterol
4-Complete multivitamin with minerals and lycopene and lutein, one daily
5-Garlic either as a fresh garlic, or supplement, but only if it can be tolerated and controlled

4. Lunch:

1-Monday-fresh broccoli, red or green bell peppers, carrots, sliced apples or pears, low salt crackers with no cholesterol and no fat. Add 2 slices of low fat cheese, like provolone. Ok to use some small amount of low fat ranch dressing to lightly dip vegetables.

2-Tuesday-same lunch, except: eliminate cheese and add tuna, white albacore in water or cooked (fresh) or baked turkey cooked with a little olive oil or lean chicken

3-Wednesday-same lunch as Tuesday

4-Thursday-same lunch as Monday

5-Friday-same lunch as Monday, except, eliminate the cheese and add tuna, or Atlantic salmon, or peanut butter

Saturday and Sunday lunches:

1-Turkey sandwich with cheese, tomato, onion, dark leafy lettuce or spinach, use mustard instead of mayonnaise or
2-Chicken sandwich or
3-Lean pork sandwich or
4-Fish sandwich

Snacks: morning between breakfast and lunch (2 hours after breakfast) and early afternoon (2 hours after lunch):

1-Fruits, sliced

2-Unsalted or low salt, fat free pretzels
3-Ryvita rye and oat bran snack crackers
4-Wasa wafers
5-Lavasch crackers, garlic flavored
6-Thin matzos unsalted crackers
7-Gold'N Krackle flatbreads-Mediterranean healthy snack food

Dinners: (Monday through Sunday)-general comments

1-Include vegetables, especially fresh or frozen fresh

2-Try to use 'non-processed' meats and meals. Fresh meats such as turkey, lean chicken, lean pork, and fish, generally have less salt, less cholesterol, and less fat

3-Breads should be healthy types, like multi-grain, flat breads and wheat and even wheat non-fat tortillas are also good

4-Red wines, especially Cabernets, are recommended

5-Always drink and prepare all foods, including teas and coffees with purified water only. Never use tap water to drink from if possible. Gallons of purified water are often cheaper than one can of soda. Also, is you drink purified water completely and you may need to supplement your daily tooth cleaning with a fluoride mouthwash

6-Desserts-try dark, semi-sweet chocolates with a cacao (cacao) solid range of 60-85%. Alternate with low fat or fat free ice cream or yogurts. Add fresh fruits and or low fat or fat free whipped creams.

7-Review all meals and where possible, add natural herbs, fruits, vegetables and healthy antioxidant drinks. Try some oxidant foods with every meal.

Here's to living a healthier, longer and happier lifestyle. Take those antioxidants, they really help.

Chapter Seven: Secret #Five-Exercise Review

At the present time, the 'fountain of youth' and the pure 'immortality pill' has yet to be found. Science is vigorously working to end disease, and prolong life, especially a healthy life. Worldwide stem cell research and new discoveries with genes and DNA are both showing encouraging possibilities for 'ultra long life'. But for now, the major conclusion is for everyone to develop a healthy lifestyle. And one of the best ways to reduce aging and possibly reverse it, is to **exercise!**

Regular physical exercise can reduce the risk of heart attacks, strokes, alzheimer's disease and even some cancers.

Why Exercise?

1. Decrease risk of having or dying from heart disease
2. Help reduce high blood pressure or the tendency to have high blood pressure
3. Help reduce high cholesterol or that tendency
4. Help reduce risk of developing colon and breast cancer
5. Help reduce risk of diabetes
6. Build and maintains more healthy muscles, bones and joints
7. Helps prevent and/or reduce depression
8. Improves feeling of well being
9. Improves self confidence
10. Improves work, sport and recreational activity
11. Improves cardiovascular endurance and maintenance function
12. Increases blood supply to brain, muscles, cells and enhances ability to utilize oxygen
13. Helps the utilization of good cholesterol, HDL
14. Helps reduce blood triglycerides
15. Helps reduce and control excess body fat
16. Improves muscle, joint, tendon and ligament strength

17. Improves balance
18. Develops brainpower at all ages
19. Helps promote better flexibility, especially for joints
20. Improves social activity

Remember, exercise not only slows aging, but some studies suggest, it may actually reverse aging! Of all the topics discussed in Kelly's Secrets, Exercise may be the most important secret so far.

How to start?

There are too many obese people, especially in America. Like or not, it's not healthy. Many professionals recommend joining an exercise spa, private club, YMCA, community recreational facility or buying your own equipment. It is also recommended that it's safer to exercise among a group and in many cases, its good social environment to see others serious about improving their health. Social exercising can be more encouraging and more motivational.

However, if exercise centers are not workable, many experts recommend purchasing a treadmill, &/or elliptical machine, &/or fitness stationary bike, and some degree of a home weight gym with dumbbells or other lifting equipment. If you decide on a home gym type set up, set up a workable goal of how much real time you plan to spend each day. That will help determine how much and what equipment to purchase or use. Many experts recommend the treadmill or elliptical as a good all around cardiovascular and general exercise machine. If the knees are an issue, the elliptical is generally recommended instead of the treadmill. But the treadmill is still a super walking machine, if running is not an option. If a elliptical is chosen, get or use one that has 'arm handles', so that you can exercise your upper body at the same time you exercise your lower body.

There are many diverse, quality **exercise machines** beyond the basic treadmill or elliptical. It may be best to review with a professional and make up your own mind. It is suggested, that when choosing, pick equipment that improves cardiovascular health first.

The other group of exercise equipment involves '**weights and stretch equipment**'. Again, with this group, the choices are practically endless. So it's very important to pick how you are going to exercise and how much time you can spend. With these types, it is recommended that you check with a professional trainer, or advisor. Remember this about your life and maybe the rest of your life, so take your time, and choose wisely. Make reachable goals based on real time.

30-60-90 rule:

Pick 30, 60 or 90 minutes a day and schedule, 5 days a week.

If you 'work too much' or cannot seem to fit this time in your schedule, consider changing your schedule. Many folks get up 30 minutes earlier and exercise in the morning before work. Although working out is beneficial whenever you can, many of those who work, prefer the mornings before breakfast and many retirees work out after breakfast and before lunch. Some folks work out after work. Whatever you choose, pick something consistent.

Before beginning any new exercise program, check with your doctor first. Let the doctor know what your are planning to do and periodically check back in with him or her. This is especially critical, if you are taking medications or have some level of disease like high blood pressure, cardiovascular issues, diabetes & other conditions. Play it safe.

One of the 'popular' choices of an exercise program is to start out slow and work up to 30, 60 or 90 minutes. But too many folks give up too soon. It may be better, to do the full 30, 60, or 90 minutes right from the start. Just start out at a slower pace and work up to more vigorous exercise.

A more balanced approach may be the best choice. For example, a good rule of thumb, is the "two-thirds" rule. 2/3 of cardiovascular exercise, for example, walking, running, stair climbing, rowing, and the last 1/3 should be used for light weights and stretching. Keep in mind that the keeping the heart healthy is the most important issue with exercise. Say, for example you choose 30 minutes a day. Then spend 20 minutes for cardio and 10 minutes with light weights and stretch. The first 20 minutes can be used to walk or run on the treadmill or used on the elliptical, and the last 10 minutes use light weights, such as dumbbells for muscle improvement and then end with some stretching for better flexibility and motion. It is also important to 'warm up' your muscles before beginning such as mild stretching.

Everyone is different, so starting out on a treadmill or elliptical or bike or combination of 2 or more can be confusing and you don't want to waste what you may be doing. So get some advice about starting out with speed, elevation and resistance. A professional advisor can help you get started the right way, based on your personal condition and abilities.

Normally, the body will resist the new work challenge until it feels more conditioned. Some folks will learn to love the exercise routine and some will not. So, it's important to make it as interesting as possible. Some exercise centers have televisions you can watch to help pass the time more quickly, some folks can read while exercising. Whatever you do, think about what you are doing. The benefits, internal and external, can be enormous. You can be proud that you are making a serious commitment to your health and life.

Should I Exercise based on Time, Speed, Distance or Calories?

Exercise is usually an individual thing. People often react differently. If you ask a person that regularly exercises, what do you base your program on? That person may often say, I work out 30 minutes a day. Or, a person may say, I work out based on burning 200-800 calories a day based on my 60-90 minute work out. Or someone may say, I run 2 miles every day.

So, it's really up to you.

Story: there was a doctor who was a member of our local community. He was (and still is) a heart surgeon. He was terribly overweight. He weighed about 300 pounds and was about 5 feet, 11 inches tall. One day, while he was conducting surgery, on one of his patients, he had an extremely sharp pain in his chest. He asked the other surgeons assisting to take over while he went to the emergency room. Fortunately, he did not have a heart attack, but he had a real warning. The next week, he joined the exercise facility and began working out with a goal of reaching 1,000 calories per day, 5 days a week. He was relentless. After 8 weeks, he reached his goal and stayed with it (and still does). He lost 140 pounds after 9 months of exercising. He now weighs around 160 and his body looks like a much younger man. His waist went from 40 to 32.

His blood pressure went from sky high to normal.

Exercise is a great way to improve and endure longer life, but it must be combined with a healthy lifestyle which includes a good diet.

Some popular exercise type machines and equipment may include:

1. Treadmill
2. Elliptical
3. Stationary fitness bike
4. Abdominal exercise machine
5. Home gyms
6. Rowing machines
7. Stepping machines
8. Stationary stretch machine

9. Yoga and Pilates kits
10. Exercise ball

The popular treadmill is a real workhorse, because of its versatile activity. One can start out slow and easy, then with professional instruction, increase speed, elevation and resistance. Most treadmills can accelerate up to speeds beyond what a normal human can run. And the elevations up to 12 or 15 can easily challenge anyone.

Working slowly and carefully, while increasing speed & elevation is important. Remember, never exercise alone.
Injuries from using some exercise equipment can be serious as well as painful, so pay attention. At the same time, it is believed by many, that holding on to the treadmill handle is not good. It may place undue stress on your lower back and spine and it is there just for temporary support. Also, not using the handle increases the exercise benefit by as much as 20%.

Walking and running are considered by some as the best form of all around exercise. Fast walking and elevated walking are also considered an excellent way to exercise. The elliptical machines are also very popular and cause less stress on the knees and joints.

Here are some simple workout schedules:

1. 30 minutes per day-20 minutes on treadmill or elliptical and 10 minutes with light weights
2. 40 minutes per day-30 minutes on treadmill or elliptical and 10 minutes with light weights
3. 60 minutes per day-40 minutes on treadmill or elliptical and 20 minutes with light weights and stretch
4. For more serious exercise: 90 minutes per day-60 minutes on treadmill and/or elliptical and 30 minutes with multiple weight activities and stretching

Light weight strength and stretch activities:

1. One of the more recent tools for lighter exercise is the use of the 'exercise ball'. It's easier on your back & spine, yet still provides some safer strength and stretching moves
2. Abdominal curl
3. Abdominal curl with twist
4. Chest press
5. Should press
6. Dumbbell curl
7. Exercise bike
8. Stand upright, bend and touch ground slowly
9. Stand upright, reach as high as you can
10. Arms behind neck, slowly turn at a 90 degree angle each way.
11. Keep in mind, that cardiovascular exercise should be done daily when you exercise. Most stomach exercises can be done daily. For lifting exercises, it may be better to alternate days for different lifts.

Diabetes-comments

Diabetes is a growing disease problem, especially in the United States. In 2005, nearly 21 million Americans (7%) had diabetes. By the year 2030, it is estimated that 30 million Americans will have the disease.

There are two types:

1. Type 2-frequently associated with older age, obesity, & also called 'adult onset', because in some cases, it may be caused due to lack of exercise. It can be prevented in majority of cases

2. Type 1-very serious, usually strikes children and young adults and accounts for 5-10% of all diagnosed cases.

Most health professionals all agree, that exercise is particularly beneficial not only to anyone with Diabetes, but in the majority of 'adult onset' type population, disease can be prevented.

Walking versus Running versus Exercise:

Quite often, many exercise rookies decide to purchase lots of equipment and or join clubs and shortly thereafter, the fad fades.

It may be more reasonable just to walk. Walking is one of the best aerobic exercises. Get a good pair of supportive, comfortable shoes and go for a walk. Many folks join a mall walking club. This is a good source of exercise and social activity. Some folks jog in a safe neighborhood community or at a school, or park or exercise facility, but remember, exercise with others. Streets and sidewalks are seldom uniform and may not be safe or flat. Many lack any security or protection. Also, exercising with someone or with a group of folks is not only more secure, but it may be more motivating and competitive.

"Nothing happens until something moves", said by Albert Einstein. Exercise develops brainpower at all ages. Movement appears to enhance memory, learning, attention, decision-making and multi-tasking. It also may slow, even reverse age-related decline. One study suggested the people who exercise, score better on mental tests than those that didn't. Also, exercise prompts structural changes in the brain of mice, spurring the growth of new nerve cells and connections between those cells. Although this was not done conclusively with human studies, finding that new neurons can be formed later in life, including old aged animals, it was promising. Scientists had long assumed that at birth we have all the nerve cells we will ever have and that as we age, we lose nerve cells. But these more recent animal studies, especially with mice, exercising helped stall the progression of dementia, helped prevent Alzheimers disease, & cognitive behavior was improved.

Aerobic exercise is exercise which is of moderate intensity and it is undertaken for a long duration. The word aerobic means with oxygen and refers to the use of oxygen in muscle energy-generating process. Aerobic exercise releases endorphins, which are your body's natural painkillers.

Even moderate exercise can improve memory and attention by 15% or more.

Ways Exercise Enhances Brain Performance:

1. Increases flow of oxygen to the brain. This may help build tiny blood vessels that pave the way for the growth of new cells.

2. Boosts substances know as growth factors: one of these, brain-derived neurotropic factor and is critical to the survival of new nerve cells.

3. Increases neurotransmitters: these brain chemicals-including dopamine, serotonin and norepinephrine play roles in cognition

Wounds Heal Faster with Exercise:

Exercise helps skin wounds on older adults heal faster (according to Charles Emery, Journal of Gerontology, Medical Sciences). The body's ability to heal, even small wounds, slows with age. But a brisk 30 to 40 minute walk ,at least three times a week, can help speed up wound healing. The mechanism is that exercise enhances the immune system.

Kelly's Favorites Regarding Exercise:

1. **Make it fun**

2. **Always do cardiovascular exercises first**

3. Begin with the hardest exercises, then work towards the easier exercises and ending with the easiest exercises, like stretching

4. After cardiovascular exercises, do any leg exercises next. Remember the legs may be 5 times stronger than the arms.

5. Drink small sips of purified water during exercise session.

6. Set goals around total calories, or time, or distance.

7. Set goals of desired weight loss and waist size reduction. Try to lose that 'belly'.

8. Never exercise alone.

9. Check with your doctor before beginning any new exercise program and check back with him or her periodically.

10. Check your blood pressure regularly.

11. Eat more slowly.

12. Do some exercise 5 times a week.

13. Choose one of the 30, 60 or 90 minute sessions.

Chapter Eight: Secret #Six-"DMVS" Dietary Minerals, Vitamins and Supplements

Back in pharmacy school, I still remember how we studied the importance of vitamins and especially how serious certain vitamin deficiencies are and they can cause disease, blindness and even death. After graduation, I began working with the public both as a pharmacist and as a manager. It was amazing how little people knew about vitamins, supplements and dietary minerals. And with the massive advertising, especially with television, newspapers and magazines, how many people can be "brainwashed" to buy these miracle television wonder drugs. Fortunately, with the immense expansion of technology, particularly with computers and internet information, anyone can look up anything, anytime and get plenty of good information, including research to help them decide which vitamins, supplements and dietary minerals to use.

The vast majority of registered pharmacists are or should be trained experts in giving good advice as to which 'DMVS', dietary minerals, vitamins and supplements, to take. Most pharmacists will give you a straight answer.

Vitamins:

When we think of vitamins, we think of them as a health additive, especially in cells, in small amounts and that they help prevent disease. Back in 1912, the word vitamin was 'coined' by a Polish biochemist, Casimir Funk. Vita, (in latin) means life, and the amin suffix is short for amine. Back then, all vitamins were thought to be amines, but that is no longer true. In 1747, Scottish surgeon, James Lind found out the citrus foods prevent scurvy (a disease marked by spongy gums, loosened teeth, and bleeding under the skin) and was caused by lack of Vitamin C. Linus Pauling, who won the Nobel prize in chemistry, always advocated taking large doses of vitamin c as a major way to enhance health and live a much longer life.

Vitamins are "organic molecules" necessary for living organisms. Deficiencies of certain vitamins will or may cause disease symptoms. There are 2 types, water soluble and fat soluble. Water soluble vitamins dissolve in water and oil soluble vitamins are absorbed via the intestinal tract with the help of lipids, which are substances, as fats and waxes, that with proteins and carbohydrates, make up the principal structural parts of living cells. Usually, an organism must obtain vitamins (or their metabolic precursors) from outside the body, mostly from the organism's diet. Examples of those that the human body can derive from precursors include Vitamin A, which can be produced from Beta-carotene, Niacin, from the amino acid, Tryptophan, and Vitamin D through exposure to sunlight (ultraviolet light).

Even ancient Egyptians knew that adding liver to a diet, would help cure night blindness, which is usually caused by Vitamin A deficiency. Throughout the early 1900's, scientists were able to isolate and identify many of the vitamins by depriving animals of them.

In humans, there are 13 basic vitamins divided in 2 groups: 4 fat soluble and 9 water soluble. All these vitamins, their uses, sources and doses will now be reviewed.

1. **Vitamin A (reinoids, include retinol, retinoic acid and 3-dehydroretinol):**

1-Fat soluble

2-Uses:

-antioxidant important in vision, bone, and tooth growth

-essential to maintenance of epithelial tissues, as a barrier to infection

-helps immune system maintenance

-helps in formation of red blood cells

-affects the production of human growth hormone

-may reduce risk of certain cancers

3-Source-sweet potatoes, collard greens, cantaloupe, pumpkin, apricots, liver, dairy products, darkly colored fruits, leafy vegetables, carrots, spinach, milk, eggs and broccoli

4-Dose: 3,500 to 10,000 units per day. Overdose can be harmful, even fatal, resulting in hypervitaminosis A and too much may also contribute to osteoporosis

2. **Vitamin B-1 Thiamin (there are 3 known: thiamin phosphate derivatives, thiamine monophosphate-thmp, thiamine diphosphate-thdp, and thiamine triphosphate-thtp**

1-Water soluble

2-Uses:

-some of the thiamine enzymes function in metabolism of carbohydrates and fats

-essential for normal growth and development and helps in functioning of the heart, nervous system and digestive system

-deficiency may cause neurodegeneration, wasting, death, and beriberi. Deficiency may also be caused by alcoholism.

3-Source: green peas, spinach, liver, beef, pork, navy beans, nuts, pinto beans, soybeans, whole grain and enriched cereals, breads, yeast, and legumes (of any large family of plants having fruits that are dry pods and split when ripe).

4-Dose: 1.5 mg per day. Some research studies have shown that daily does of 50 mg, have shown to increase mental activity. Overdose: only known cases of thiamin overdose occurred with thiamin injection, causing anaphylactic reaction.

3. Vitamin B-2 Riboflavin

1-Water soluble

2-Uses:

-key role in health in animals especially growth

-aids in metabolism of fats, carbohydrates, and proteins

-required for red blood cell formation, respiration, antibody production, regulation of human growth hormone and reproduction

-essential for healthy skin, nails, hair growth and general good health, including regulation of thyroid activity

-helps prevent many eye disorders, including some cases of cataracts

-helps when eyes are bloodshot, or have abnormal sensitivity to light

-deficiency, called ariboflavinosis may cause cracked and red lips, inflammation of the lining of mouth, tongue, mouth ulcers, cracks at corner of mouth, and sore throat. Also, dry and scaly skin, fluid in mucous membranes, and iron deficiency anemia. In animals, deficiency results in lack of growth, failure to thrive and eventual death. Excess causes urine to turn bright yellow.

3-Source: milk, cheese, leafy green vegetables, liver, yeast, almonds, mature soybeans

4-Dose: 1.7 mg per day

4. **Vitamin B-3 Niacin (also known as nicotinic acid and in amide form, niacinamide)**

1-Water soluble

2-Uses:

-plays essential roles in energy metabolism in living cells and DNA repair

-role in production of several sex and stress related hormones, especially those made by the adrenal gland

-helps remove toxic and harmful chemicals from the body

-helps terminate a 'bad trip' on LSD (Lysergic-diethylamide)

-helps, in large doses, to increase level of high density lipoprotein (HDL) or good cholesterol in blood

-popular belief that it can be used to mask marijuana use in urine tests, but scientific evidence is not available

-used as a food additive, typically to improve color of ground meat

-important for normal health of digestive tract, skin, nerves and brain

-deficiencies, called "pellagra" may cause skin rash, disease of digestive system and nervous symptoms

3-Source: liver, heart and kidney, chicken, beef, fish, tuna, salmon, milk, eggs, leafy vegetables, broccoli, tomatoes, carrots, dates, sweet potatoes, asparagus, avocados, nuts, whole grain products, legumes, saltbush seeds, mushrooms, and brewer's yeast

4-Dose: 20 mg/day   high dose=100mg

5. Vitamin B-5 Pantothenic acid

1-Water soluble

2-Uses:

-required to sustain life

-needed to form co-enzyme-A (COA). Co-enzyme A is thought to assist in the transport of carbon atoms within the cell, by helping in cellular respiration as well as the biosynthesis of many important compounds such as fatty acids, cholesterol and acetylcholine

-critical in the metabolism and synthesis of carbohydrates, proteins and fats

-considered essential in all forms of life

-deficiency is called 'paresthesia' and pantothenic acid deficiency is very rare. Victims of starvation have been noted and symptoms are similar to other vitamin b deficiencies. Some minor symptoms reported are fatigue, allergies, nausea and abdominal pain

3-Source: small amounts are found in most foods with high quantities in whole grain and eggs. Also found in many dietary supplements and in some energy drinks. Also may be generated in humans from gut bacteria

4-Dose: 5-10 mg per day

6. Vitamin B-6 Pyridoxine (also called pyridoxal, pyridoxamine)

1-Water soluble

2-Uses:

-assists in balancing of sodium (na) and potassium (k) as well as promoting red blood cell production

-helps in cardiovascular health by decreasing the formation of homocysteine

-helps children with learning difficulties

-helps prevent dandruff, eczema, and psoriasis

-helps balance hormonal changes in women and aid in immune system

-aids in treatment of depression and anxiety

-helps maintain healthy nerve and muscle cells and aids in production of DNA and RNA

-it is necessary for proper absorption of vitamin B-12 (Cyanocobalamin)
-'woman's vitamin', because it helps relieve symptoms of premenstrual syndrome (pms)

-considered anti-stress vitamin because enhances immune system

-helps people with burns

-helps control blood sugar with those who have diabetes

-helps energy conversion

-promotes healthy nerves and muscles

-deficiency causes anemia, nerve damage, irritability, depression, difficulty with concentration and short term memory loss

3-Source: dragon fruit (south east Asia), chicken, turkey, tuna, salmon, shrimp, beef liver, lentils, soybeans, nuts, avocados, bananas, carrots, brown rice, bran, sunflower seeds, wheat germ and whole grain flour

4-Dose: 2 mg per day   upper level is 100 mg per day

7. Vitamin B-7 Biotin (also known as Vitamin H)

1-Water soluble

2-Uses:

-important in the catalysis of essential metabolic reactions to synthesize fatty acids

-helps prevent hair loss in children and adults. Severe deficiency include loss of eye lashes and eye brows

-in diabetes, type 2, low levels of biotin may exist

-may be involved in the synthesis and release of insulin

-may improve blood sugar control in those with type 2 diabetes
-used in cell growth

-plays a role in the Krebs cycle (process where energy is released from food)

-helps in transfer of carbon dioxide

-helps maintain steady level of blood sugar

-helps strengthen hair and nails

-deficiency is rare, but can become very serious, even fatal if not treated. Deficiency may cause dry skin, seborrheic dermatitis, fungal infections, rashes, fine and brittle hair, hair loss (or total 'alopecia'), mild depression, changes in mental status, muscular pain (myalgias)

3-Sources: liver, kidney, some seafood, especially oysters, lobster and salmon, yeast, cauliflower, chicken breast, egg yolk (not egg white)

4-Dose: 30-300 micrograms (mcg or ug)

8. Vitamin B-9 Folic Acid (folate)

1-Water soluble

2-Uses:

-nutrient needed to prevent anemia during pregnancy

-necessary for production and maintenance of new cells, especially periods of rapid cell division and growth such as infancy and pregnancy

-needed to replicate DNA

-helps prevent changes to DNA that may lead to cancer

-helps both adults and children make normal red blood cells and prevent anemia

-helps prevent against congenital malformation including spine bifida, skull and brain (anencephaly)

-can help correct anemia associated with B-12 deficiency, but the cause of B-12 deficiency must be corrected. Back in 1996, the FDA (food and drug administration) published regulations to add folic acid to enriched breads, cereals, flours, corn meals, pastas, rice and other grain products, targeted to reduce birth defects in newborns

-deficiencies may hinder DNA synthesis and cell division, affecting bone marrow, a site of rapid cell turnover. And may cause megaloblastic anemia; low concentrations may increase risk for heart disease and stroke due to elevated homocysteine. Also some evidence that low levels of folate (folic acid) may increase risk of cancer

3-Source: leafy vegetables, spinach, turnip greens, dried beans and peas, fortified cereals, sunflower seeds, and other fruits and vegetables

4-Dose: 400 mcg/day (micrograms) upper dose level 1,000 mcg

9. Vitamin B-12 Cyanocobalamin

1-Water soluble

2-Uses:
-helps prevent several forms of anemia

-used in treatment of cyanide poisoning

-helps maintain cardiovascular and nerve health

-helps produce normal red blood cells

-deficiencies can cause several forms of anemia, especially megaloblastic anemia and pernicious anemia. Excessive alcohol intake, certain antibiotics, bc pills, and many other drugs decrease B-12 absorption. Proton pump inhibitors (ppi's), such as Prilosec (omeprazole), Prevacid (lansprazole), Aciphex (rabeprazole), Prontonix, Pantoloc (pantoprazole) and Nexium (esomeprazole), all may reduce the absorption of B-12
.

-dermatologic reactions: itching, rash, transatory exantherma and uticaria. There have been some research suggesting that combination doses of B-12 20 mcg or more plus Pyridoxine (B-6), 80 mg or more may cause symptoms of Rosacea. Also, Metformin (glucophagel) , Neomycin, nicotine, nitrous oxide, Phenytoin (Dilantin), phenobarbital, primidone (Mysoline) may also decrease absorption of B-12.

3-Source: meats, especially liver & shellfish, eggs, milk products, fortified cereals, fortified soy-based products, fortified energy bars

4-Dose: 2.4 mcg (micrograms) daily western diet 5-7 mcg

10. Vitamin C Ascorbic Acid

1-Water soluble

2-Uses:

-nature's most powerful and safest antioxidant

-prevents scurvy (disease with spongy gums, loosened teeth, bleeding under the skin)

-protects body cells from potential oxidative damage and enhances the immune system

-safest vitamin known

-helps prevent stroke, cancer and hypertension

-helps prevent colds

-helps prevent heart diseases

-helps to treat viral diseases due to antihistamine effect

-helps to treat many poisons

-may help prevent cataract formation

-most widely used as a dietary supplement

-improves blood vessel and cardiovascular integrity

-enhances healthy hormone actions

-enhances nitrous oxide functions

-rebuilds the powerful antioxidant, glutathione

-improves intestinal transit time

-reduces the accumulation of toxins

-protects our DNA from damage

-reduces toxic minerals in the body

-rebuilds Vitamin E and Selenium

-maintains the integrity of cartilage, bones and teeth

-increases cellular resistance to many common viral infections

-overall increase in energy and improved sense of well being

3-Source: found in citrus fruits, cherries, cantaloupe, strawberries, vegetables, especially red and green, peppers, broccoli, brussels sprouts, tomatoes, asparagus, parsley, dark leafy greens and cabbage, oranges and orange juice, grapefruit and grapefruit juice

4-Dose: 500-3,000 mg per day upper level dose 2,000 mg/day. Some cases may suggest 'mega doses', such as several thousand mg/day

11. Vitamin D's

Vitamin D-1= molecular compound of ergo calciferol with innoisterol

Vitamin D-2= ergo calciferol or calciferol

Vitamin D-3 =cholecalciferol, made from 7-dehydrocholesterol in the skin

Vitamin D-4 =dihydrotachysterol

Vitamin D-5=sitocalciferol, made from 7-dehydrocholesterol in the skin

Vitamin D's are a group of fat soluble 'pro-hormones', the two major forms of which are **Vitamin D-2 (ergocalciferol) and Vitamin D-3 (or cholecalciferol).** D's also refer to metabolites and other analogues of these substances. D-3 is produced in skin exposed to sunlight, specifically ultraviolet 'b' radiation. Very few foods are naturally rich in Vitamin D, and most Vitamin D intake is in the form of fortified products including milk, soy milk and cereal grains.

Vitamin D's also regulate the calcium and phosphorus levels in the blood by promoting their absorption from food in the intestines and by promoting re-absorption of calcium in the kidneys.

1-Fat soluble

2-Uses:
-D's promote bone formation and mineralization and is essential in the development of an intact and strong skeleton

-inhibit parathyroid hormone secretions from the parathyroid gland

-affects the immune system by promoting immunosuppression and anti-tumor activity

-found to induce death of cancer cells

-deficiency may cause liver or kidney disorders, impaired bone mineralization, bone softening diseases, such as rickets in children and osteomalacia in adults and possibly contribute to osteoporosis

3-Source: fish liver oils, fatty fish (salmon, mackerel, sardines, tuna), whole eggs, shiitake mushrooms

4-Dose: 5-10 mcg (micrograms)   upper levels 50 mcg severe overdose may cause gi symptoms, anorexia, nausea and vomiting, polyuria (passage of large volume of urine), polydipsia (increase in thirst) and even renal failure

12. Vitamin E Tocopherol

Alpha Tocopherol is the only form of Vitamin E that is actively maintained in the human body and appears to be the most significant as an antioxidant.

1-Fat soluble

2-Uses:

-main use is to be an antioxidant and therefore intercept free radicals and prevent a chain reaction of lipid destruction

-helps maintain cell membranes throughout the body

-reduces risk of heart related deaths including cardiac arrest by at least 24%

-may help cut the risk of prostate cancer by 50%

-helps reduce formation of cataracts

-helps cut risk of 'ALS' (Lou Gehrigs Disease) by 64%

-helps reduce risk of cancer by preventing free radical damage

-helps fight alzheimers

-helps fight macular degeneration

-helps fight infections, colds, flu and low immunity

-may reduce other types of cardiovascular disease

-may help reduce risk or affect of dementia (impaired cognitive function)

3-Source: vegetable oils, like olive, sunflower, and safflower oils, also in nuts, whole grains, and green leafy vegetables

4-Dose: adult range 200-1,500 units daily, average supplement range 400-600 IU (international units)

13. Vitamin K Naphthoquinone

There are two forms of Vitamin k-1, Phylloquinone and Vitamin k-2, Menaquinones

1-Fat soluble

2-Uses:

-Vitamin K (Kougulation) is essential for the functioning of several proteins in blood clotting

-helps to prevent the calcification of soft tissues and cartilage

-facilitates normal bone growth and development

-cellular growth regulation factors are associated with Vitamin K

-plays a role in the development and aging of the nervous system

-deficiency results in impaired blood clotting, and may result in nosebleeds, bleeding gums, blood in the urine, blood in the stools, black stools, or extremely heavy menstrual bleeding and in infants, deficiency may result in intracranial hemorrhage

3-Source: naturally occurs in alfalfa, green leafy vegetables, vegetable oils, such as soybean, cottonseed, canola, and olive. Also in broccoli, spinach, and mayonnaise

4-Dose: 100-120 mcg/day older adults (65 and older) are at increase risk of osteoporosis and hip fracture, some studies suggest a daily dose of 250 mcg/day and one cup of dark green leafy vegetables daily

Non-Vitamin, "Vitamins"

1. Vitamin F-originally given to essential fatty acids that the body cannot manufacture. They were de-vitaminized, because they are fatty acids. Fatty acids are a major component of fats which, like water, are needed by the body in large quantities and thus do not fit the definition of vitamins which are needed only in trace amounts

2. Vitamin T, vitamin U and vitamin X-herbalists and naturopaths may have called these therapedic chemicals, vitamins, but they are not

3. Ubiquinone or Coenzyme Q-10 is manufactured in small amounts by the body, like Vitamin D, but it is not a vitamin

4. Vitamin B-15 or Pangamic acid, is a related substance, dimethylglycine, but it is not a vitamin and is also referred to as B-16

5. Vitamin B-17 is really laetrile and/or amyglydine. B-17 anti-cancer properties have been disproven by many experiments

6. Vitamin P- Flavanoids are sometimes called vitamin P

7. Vitamin B-10-some animal, bird and bacterial growth factors have been designated 'vitamins'. Examples of these are 'para-aminobenzoic acid (paba)' and folacin (see folic acid) pteryl-hepta-glutamic acid which is the chicken feathering factor called 'Vitamin-11'.

8. B-4 (adenine) and B-8 (adenylic acid) in the past were thought to be part of b-complex vitamins, but later it was found that this is not true.

"Slang" Vitamins-Common Vitamin Word(s) Used to Denote A Certain Vitamin or Type of Vitamin:

1. Vitamin A-slang word referring to alcoholic beverage

2. Vitamin C-slang word used to refer to caffeine

3. Vitamin G-slang word for Guinness

4. Vitamin H-refers to Biotin

5. Vitamin I-refers to ibuprofen

6. Vitamin J-refers to Jagermeister, a herbal German liquor

7. Vitamin K-refers to the sedative, Ketamine which is used as a recreational drug

8. Vitamin Love-refers to Patti Page's song, "I don't care if the sun don't shine"

9. Vitamin W-refers to water

10. Vitamin V-refers to Viagra

11. Vitamin Z-refers to Zoloft

12. Vitamin R-refers to Ritalin

Dietary Minerals (human intake)

Dietary minerals are **chemical elements** required by living organisms, other than carbon, hydrogen, nitrogen and oxygen which are everywhere in organic molecules. Remember, that **Vitamins** are **organic molecules** necessary for living organisms, especially cells.

Dietary minerals can be either **bulk**, (need large amounts) or **trace** (only small amounts needed). Also, we will review several "other minerals" which have some significant properties.

1. Dietary minerals include, Calcium, Magnesium,

Phosphorous, Potassium, Sodium, Sulfur and Chlorine.

2. Trace minerals include, Chromium, Cobalt, Copper,

Fluorine, Iodine, Iron, Manganese, Molybdenum, Selenium,

And Zinc.

3. "Other Minerals" include:

Bismuth, Boron, Nickel, Rubidium, Silicon, Strontium,

Tellurium, Titanium, Tungsten, Vanadium

4. Other supplements include:

Lutein, Lycopene, Tin, Omega-3 fatty acid, Co-Enzyme (c0q10),

Hgh (human growth hormone), St. John's Wort, Garlic,

Inositol, Paba, and Choline.

Upon first looking at these minerals and supplements, it looks like, oh no, not another chemistry lesson! Not really, this review homes in on how these minerals can help us all live a lot longer and a lot healthier. Many of these minerals are not only pure life saving, but many actually allow life to exist. We will cover bulk minerals first.

Bulk minerals:

Some of these are naturally occurring in food or can be added in elemental or mineral form such as calcium carbonate or sodium chloride (salt). Proper intake levels of each dietary mineral must be sustained to maintain physical health. Excesses can harm the body. We will try to review those bulk minerals, trace minerals and other minerals and supplements as they relate to human health, and longevity.

1. Calcium (ca):

1-Uses: essential in muscle contraction, oocyte activation, bones and tooth structure, blood clotting, nerve impulse transmission, heartbeat regulation and fluid balance within all cells. In the United States, 50-75% of adults do not get enough calcium in their diet.

2-Sources: milk, cheese, seaweeds, nuts, seeds (especially almonds & sesame), molasses, beans, oranges, collard greens, broccoli, okra, and soymilk

3-Dose: adults need between 1,000-1,300 mg of calcium dialy.

2. Magnesium (mg):

1-Uses: contributes to the tartness and taste of natural waters, essential for strong teeth and bones, used as an ionic laxative, used as a mild base, used as an antacid, used as magnesium sulfate as 'Epsom salts'. Ion form is essential to the basic nucleic chemistry of life and essential to all cells of all known organisms. Used in manufacture of fireworks, and marine flares, used in the synthesis of DNA and RNA. Deficiency associated with muscle spasms, cardiovascular disease, diabetes, high blood pressure, anxiety disorders, and osteoporosis. Also used to treat hypertension of eclampsia and in the citrate form, used as a laxative known as "milk of magnesia"

2-Sources: green vegetables (especially spinach), nuts (especially almonds), seeds, and some whole grains

3-Dose: 400mg/ day. An overdose may cause diarrhea, and disturbed nervous system function

3. Phosphorous (p)

1-Uses: it is a component of DNA and RNA and is an essential element for all living cells, used in food applications such as soda beverages and baking powder, helps improve characteristics of processed meat and cheese, helps improve characteristics of toothpaste, part of the main structural components of all cellular membranes, and plays an important role in bone health

2-Source: not found free in nature due to its reactivity with air and other substances. Important source is 'phosphate rock'

3-Dose: supplement range is usually 48-109 mg/day which is about 5-11% of daily value. Usual daily need is around 1,000 mg/ day

4. Potassium (k)

1-Uses: essential for proper nerve and muscle function, essential element for all living organisms, salt substitute and is used in surgery to stop the heart and in execution, by lethal injection. In the superoxide form, K0-2, source of portable oxygen, used as food preservative, except in meats. Used in baking powder and medicine, essential mineral macronutrient in human nutrition and important in maintaining fluid and electrolyte balance in the body. Shortage in the body fluids can cause death. Diets high in potassium can reduce risk of hypertension

2-Source: orange juice, bananas, potatoes, avocados, apricots, fruits and vegetables, and meats

3-Dose: usual daily need may be around 3,500 mg/day. Supplements provide about 80-100mg or 2% of dietary value

5. Sodium (na) exists mostly as sodium chloride or salt

1-Uses: sodium ions are necessary for regulation of blood and body fluids, transmission of nerve impulses, heart activity, and certain metabolic functions. Extra sodium may cause an increase in blood pressure. Sodium ions also play a critical role in the human central nervous system, and in extracellular fluids, such as plasma and other tissues, sodium bathe cells and carry out transport functions for nutrients and wastes

2-Source: salt, or sodium chloride

3-Dose: human requirement is only 500 mg/day and the average American, may consume 10 times that daily.

6. Sulfur:

Sulfur is used to help skin rashes, eczema, laxatives, and is essential in all living cells

7. Chlorine:

Chlorine (usually as the chloride) is used in the formation of many every day items and to purify water. It is also necessary to human life. The chloride daily value is about 72mg.

Trace Minerals (only small amounts needed):

1. Chromium:

Chromium plays a role in metabolism of carbohydrates, proteins and fats.

Dose: 120 mcg

2. Cobalt:

Cobalt is used in many medical applications especially in radiotherapy and dental. It is essential to human life and is the central component of vitamin B-12, Cobalamin. Daily dose of B-12 is 6 mcg.

3. Copper:

Copper is essential for red blood cell formation. Dose is 2 mg/day

4. Fluorine:

Fluorine is used in dental fluorides to prevent dental cavities and to make fluorodated water. It is also used in anesthesia, anti-fungal drugs, anti-depressants and in radio-isotopes

5. Iodine:

Iodine is important for proper thyroid function. Dose 150 mcg

6. Iron:

Iron is important for production of red blood cells. Dose is 18 mg

7. Manganese:

Manganese plays a role in skeletal development and maintenance. Dose is 2 mg

8. Molybdenum:

Molybdenum functions as a cofactor for enzymes that trigger chemical reactions. Dose 75 mcg

9. Selenium (se):

Selenium is a natural part of antioxidant enzymes that help protect cells from oxidation. It also plays a role in thyroid function. Dose is 20 mcg (29 % of daily value)

10. Zinc (zn):

Zinc is an essential component of many enzymes involved in digestion, metabolism and reproduction. It also protects against premature aging of skin and muscles. In larger doses, it may help speed up the healing process after injury, and is used in throat lozenges or tablets to help remedy the common cold. It is also an essential element, needed to sustain cell life. Dose is 15 mg

Other minerals:

1. Bismuth:

Bismuth is used in cosmetic preparations.

2. Boron:

Boron is used in some compounds and shows promise in treating arthritis. Dose 150 mcg

3. Nickel:

Nickel has various roles in human biology. Dose is 5 mcg * (*=daily value, not established)

4. Rubidium:

Rubidium is used in radioactive isotopes.

5. Silicon:

Silicon is an essential element in the body. Used in breast implants, contact lenses. Dose 2 mg *

6. Strontium:

Strontium is a radio pharmaceutical used for bone pain in metastatic prostate cancer and other cancer therapies. It is also used in some toothpastes

7. Tellurium:

Tellurium is used in radio isotopes and in compounds with gold and silver.

8. Titanium:

Titanium is used in toothpastes, surgical and dental implants, joint replacements, body piercing, and golf equipment.

9. Tungsten:

Tungsten is used in shielding in radiopharmaceuticals, and nuclear medicine.

10. Vanadium:

Vanadium is an essential element in some enzymes. Some compounds help alleviate diabetes mellitus and is used as a mineral health supplement. Dose 10 mcg *

Other supplements:

1. Lutein:

Lutein is an antioxidant, also has health benefits to the eye, especially the retina. Dose 250 mcg *

2. Lycopene:

Lycopene is one of the most potent carotenoid antioxidants. It helps quence singlet oxygen, helps prevent skin aging, reduces risk of cardiovascular disease, cancer, especially prostate cancer. It also helps prevent diabetes, osteoporosis, male infertility, reduces risk of esophageal, colorectal and oral cancer. Dose 300 mcg *

3. Tin (sn):

Tin is used in food preservation, and is an important salt as stannous fluoride to prevent dental decay. Dose 10 mcg *

4. Omega-3 fatty acid or fish oil omega-3 supplement:

Omega-3 fatty acids are a family of poly unsaturated fatty acids (pfa). There are three and they are: linolenic acid, eicosapentaenoic acid, and docosahexaenoic acid.

Omega-3's are essential to normal growth in young children and in supporting dermal integrity, renal function, parturition (childbirth). They are also important in biological functions including synthesis from fatty acids and ending with metabolism by enzymes. They also reduce the risk of coronary heart disease, help in treatment of autism and help enhance membrane capabilities in brain cells. Dose is 1-3 grams/day, with 3 grams considered maximum.

5. Co-Enzyme (coq10) also known as 'Ubiquinone'

Recently, Co-Enzyme, COq10, has been used as a supplement to help reduce the risk of heart attacks, especially to those taking statin drugs to reduce cholesterol because the statins have a side effect of blocking production of co-enzyme. It is naturally synthesized in the body and plays an essential role in the production of cellular energy, especially for the heart.

Co-enzyme, coq10, also, may help our immune systems and reduce periodontal disease, cancer and aids. It is also an antioxidant by reducing plaque formation by protecting low density lipoproteins (LDL), "lousy (low) cholesterol". Dose is ranged between 10-150 mg daily *(daily value not established)

6. "HGH" Human Growth Hormone (Somatropin)

This hormone is very controversial to say the least. It is claimed to be an 'anti-aging' therapy, but real proof remains to be substantiated. Since this particular supplement's use is somewhat questionable, we will review in more detail.

Human growth hormone, Somatropin or 'HGH',is an amino acid hormone stored in the pituitary gland. Its function is to stimulate growth and cell production in humans. Growth hormone anti-aging claims were based on several reports, one reporting that all the men had significant increases in lean body mass and bone material. Other studies, showed healthy elderly patients increased muscle mass by two kilograms and decreased body fat by the same amount. However, some researchers didn't find any muscle gain, and believed that the growth hormone just lets the body store more water in muscles, rather than increase in muscle strength.

Regular use of a growth hormone, did cause joint swelling, joint pain, carpal tunnel syndrome and an increased risk of diabetes. Other side effects of growth hormone may include:

1-Swelling of the hands and feet (edema)

2-Thickening of the bones and jaws

3-Carpal tunnel syndrome and arthralgia (joint pain)

4-Tingling in the extremities

5-Numbness in the hands and feet

6-Increased organ growth

7-Decreased insulin reception

8-Acromegaly (extremity enlargement)

9-Decreased thyroid output

Growth hormone may be more dangerous to cancer sufferers, or to individuals with an increased chance of cancer, especially smokers, and may increase their mortality rate.

Human Growth Hormone "Quackery":

If growth hormone was a real fountain of youth, it would be the most powerful 'Vitamin of Health' in the world. Here are some of the growth hormone **claims to fame:**

1-Sheds body fat

2-Increases muscle tone

3-Boost energy, strength, and endurance

4-Reduces wrinkles and creates tighter, smoother skin

5-Helps you sleep better

6-Improves sex drive and performance

7-Improves immune and heart function, bone density, healing time and cholesterol

8-Improves brain function, memory and mental focus

Actual Functions of Growth Hormone:

Actual effects of growth hormone on the tissues of the body are really 'Anabolic", meaning building up:

1-Helps in growth of long bones, and cartilage of children

2-Other growth-stimulating effects on a wide variety of tissues

3-Increase in growth height

4-Increase in calcium retention, strengthens and increases bone mineralization

5-Increases in muscle mass by creating new muscle cells

6-Promotes lipolysis, which reduces body fat

7-Increases protein synthesis and stimulates growth of all internal organs including the brain

8-Reduces liver uptake of glucose (opposite of insulin)

9-Promotes liver gluconeogenesis

10-Plays a role in fuel homeostasis (equilibrium state)

11-Contributes to maintenance and function of pancreatic islets

12-Stimulates the immune system

Growth Hormone Problems: Too Much or Too Little:

Excess: (Acromegaly and Pituitary Gigantism)

1-Cells of pituitary (adenoma) may become larger and cause headaches, impaired vision or cause deficiency in pituitary hormones

2-Thickens bones of jaws, fingers and toes resulting in a heaviness

3-Pressure on nerves (carpal tunnel), muscle weakness, insulin resistance, type-2 diabetes, and reduced sexual function

4-Growth secreting tumors

Deficiency: (GHD)

1-Growth failure and short stature

2-Deficiencies of strength, energy, bone mass and increase risk of cardiovascular issues

Therapeutic uses of growth hormone:

1-Growth hormone deficiency, including shortness (turner syndrome)

2-Chronic renal failure

3-Prader-Willi Syndrome (genetic disorder due to missing genes resulting in smaller stature and learning difficulties)

4-Intrauterine growth retardation

5-Improve height, muscle strength, body fat reduction, and increase muscle mass (especially with aids)

6-Short bowel syndrome

Controversial Uses with Growth Hormone:

1-Reverse effects of aging in older adults

2-Increase weight loss in obesity

3-Treat Fibromyalgia (chronic syndrome with joint, muscle, and bone pain and fatigue)

4-Treat Crohn's disease (inflammatory bowel disorder), and ulcerative colitis

5-Treat short stature

6-Treat for body-building or athletic enhancement

7. St. John's Wort

St. John's Wort is a herbal plant (herpericum perforatum) also called 'klamath' or 'goat weed'. It is poisonous to grazing livestock, and is used as an external anti-inflammatory, astringent, and as an antiseptic. Internally, it is used to treat depression and anxiety disorders. The dose ranges from 350-1800mg per day for clinical depression, but there is a potential for drug interaction, especially with other anti-depressant agents

8. Garlic Supplement

Garlic Uses:

1-May support healthy heart function and help reduce excess cholesterol

2-Crushed raw garlic is strongly antibiotic and has a reputation of lowering blood pressure, although some studies have not proven this.

3-Powerful and popular cooking companion

4-Used as a palliative in the heat of the sun

5-May benefit those with smallpox, dropsy and tuberculosis

6-Some studies suggest benefit in treatment of hyper-cholesterol, but firm positive results may be questionable

7-Some reports relate that garlic helps in preventing and fighting the common cold.

8-May also possess some cancer-fighting properties

9-May help in healing wounds and even help prevent the onset of gangrene

10-Other uses include treatment for intestinal worms, and other internal parasites, chest infections, digestive disorders and fungal infections (thrush) and even vaginal yeast infections.

Dose range is usually about 650mg/day, but 'daily value' has not been established.

9. "Paba" Para-Aminobenzoic Acid

Paba is used in sunscreens, helps with the formation of folic acid, hair growth and protein metabolism. Sources include: liver, kidney, brewer's yeast, whole grains, mushrooms and spinach. Dose is 50 mg/day

10. Choline

Choline is an essential nutrient and is used in lipid metabolism, and it helps reduce body fat, decrease heart disease, decrease cholesterol, increase cognition, improves brain functions and is used in cellular membrane composition and repair. Sources include, beef liver, egg yolks, soy, cauliflower, celery, lettuce, peanuts, peanut butter and sunflower seeds.
Dose range is around 550mg/ day

Kelly's Favorites: "DMVS" Dietary Minerals, Vitamins and Supplements:

1. **Complete Multivitamin for adults with all Vitamins plus Dietary Minerals and Trace Elements**

2. Vitamin C 1500-2,000 mg per day, time release

3. Vitamin D 400 units with calcium 600mg-1,200 mg per day

4. Vitamin E capsules 400 units per day

5. Omega-3 fish oil enteric coated tablets or capsules 1,000 mg, 2-3 times daily

6. Joint Therapy-with Glucosamine, 1,500mg, MSM (methylsulfonylmethane) 1,500mg and Chondroitin sulfate 200 mg plus Proprietary Extract 250mg, and Hyaluronic acid (joint fluid) 3.3 mg dose range is usually 3 per day

7. Olive oil-use olive oil on salads and breads and to cook with

8. Garlic-use fresh raw garlic to cook with meals and use as much as you can tolerate.

Chapter Nine: Secret #Seven-Special Reports and Reviews Including Some of Kelly's Favorites

This chapter contains condensed summaries of many popular, and interesting articles regarding extreme longevity, and superior health tips.

1. "Kelly's Favorites" Want To Live to Be a 100 or Longer?

1-Ease up on your grump quotient-you and everyone around you might live longer

2-Try sticking to a plant based diet

3-Stay active and with a lower calorie diet

4-Share work and worries with spouse

5-Keep the faith

6-Avoid junk food and excess caffeine

7-Eat Pecorino cheese (Italian cheese from sheep's milk)

8-Drink red wine in moderation-Cabernet red's may be the healthiest

9-Eat more Red Vegetables (Red Vegetables and Wine have more antioxidants and prolong life)

10-Don't smoke, especially cigarettes. You may lose up to 10-15 years of potential living and the certain end of which may be most debilitating, leading to possible emphysema, cancer and death

11-Keep socially engaged. Social interaction is healthy and stimulating and can prolong life

12-Eat fruits, vegetables and whole grains with as many meals as possible

13-Eat nuts (non-salted are the most healthy), especially walnuts, almonds, hazel nuts and pecans

14-Eat beans-healthy and have protein and fiber

15-Keep life long friends

16-Eat more slowly, enjoy eating

17-Eat smaller portions and share bigger meals

18-Find purpose-retirement should and can easily be "planned". Hobbies and activities should be organized, interesting and balanced

19-Learn to play a musical instrument or a new language or new sport

20-Seniors who live near loved ones tend to live longer

21-Good vegetables, like zucchini, eggplant, tomatoes, fava beans ('vicia' beans that may help reduce and prevent hypertension and also help to prevent and treat parkinson disease) help reduce risk of heart disease and colon cancer

22-Good genes help a lot, but a strong healthy lifestyle with a healthy diet and exercise can be just as important if not more

23-Daily exercise is one good reason for living

24-Eat fish up to twice a week.

25-Have a strong sense of purpose buffers against stress, and disease such as hypertension

26-Herbs, spices, fruits and vegetables such as Chinese radishes, garlic, scallions, cabbage, turmeric and tomatoes contain compounds that may block cancers before they start

27-Eat sweet potatoes, carrots, bananas and drink skim milk

28-Regular churchgoers appear to live as much as 2 years longer than non-churchgoers

29-Take time off

30-Eat whole grain breads and rolls

31-Drink five glasses of purified water per day and 4 servings of nuts per week, reduces risk of heart disease

32-Take very good care of your teeth and your gums. Brush and floss, twice a day. There is strong evidence that good dental care can help improve health and reduce risk of heart and other diseases.

33-Some studies suggest no meat days and supplement with fish and/ or cheese.

2. Is It Possible To Live To Be 150?

Aubrey De Grey, Biogerontologist, says 'radical increases in life expectancy will become possible in the next 30 years', and "As medicine becomes more powerful, we will inevitably be able to address aging just as effectively as we address many diseases today". By using a special fixable technology, it should be possible to keep people alive up to age 150.

One study suggests, that aging of the 'whole organism' is caused by seven types of molecular or cellular damage. This aging damage is potentially fixable by technology that already exists today. This technology is in active development and is called 'Transhumanism'.

Transhumanism is an international intellectual and cultural movement supporting the use of new sciences and technologies to enhance human mental and physical abilities and aptitudes, and ameliorate what it regards as undesirable and unnecessary aspects of human condition, such as stupidity, suffering, disease, **aging,** and involuntary death.

Aging is the declining ability to respond to stress, including homeostatic (maintenance of stable state of equilibrium between interrelated physiological, psychological or social factors unique to an individual) imbalance and risk of disease. Therefore, death is the ultimate consequence of aging. Differences in maximum life span between species correspond to different rates of aging. Genetic inheritance makes a mouse elderly at 3 years and a human elderly at 90 years. These genetic differences are related to:

1. Efficiency of DNA (deoxy-ribonuclecic acid) repair

2. Antioxidant enzymes

3. Rates of free radical production

3. DNA, RNA, Genes, Chromosomes and Mitochondrial DNA-What Are They?

1. DNA: deoxyribonucleic acid, is a coiled threadlike molecule that conveys genetic information based on an alphabet of four building blocks called nucleotides. A gene consists of a sequence of nucleotides.

2. Genes: a gene is a specific stretch of DNA with instructions for a particular inherited characteristic, usually a protein. A gene's sequence is organized so that units of three nucleotides specify particular components in a protein. To make a protein, the DNA unwinds, exposing the gene sequence to copying enzymes. Together genes act as a recipe for building an organism.

3. RNA: ribonucleic acid, is a structure similar to DNA. Different forms do different jobs inside the cell: like copying a gene's sequence from the DNA, or carrying the message to other cell parts, or making proteins from those instructions. Viruses for flu, aids, and some other diseases have no DNA. Their genes are made of RNA.

4. Chromosomes: chromosomes are the compressed 'x' shaped structures that form when strands of DNA coil up tightly just before a cell divides. Chromosomes come in pairs, one from each parent. Each person inherits 23 pairs.

5. Mitochondrial DNA: mitochondrial DNA is a distinct type of DNA inside the mitochondria, the capsule-shaped powerhouses of cells. Scientists think mitochondria have their own DNA because they were once free-living organisms.

4. Low Dose Aspirin Daily Therapy!

Many studies recommend that folks over 40 or 50 should take enteric coated, 81 mg aspirin everyday. The primary reason seems to be to help prevent against heart attacks and possibly help reduce the risk of colon cancer. However, if you drink alcohol, like 2 or more drinks a day, if may be advised not to take daily low dose aspirin and the same may be true with other anti-inflammatory pain killers. Acetaminophen may not be a good alternative, because in large doses, it may cause liver damage.

5. "Grape Expectations"-Resveratrol, Powerful Antioxidant

Resveratrol (trans-3, 5, 4-trihydroxystilbene) is a compound found largely in the skin of red grapes. It is a compound of Ko-Jo-Kon, an oriental medicine used to treat diseases of the blood vessels, heart and liver. It came to the scientific attention around 1995 as a possible explanation of the "French Paradox"=low incidence of heart disease among the French people, who eat a relatively high-fat diet. It is touted as an antioxidant, anti-cancer agent.

While present in other plants such as eucalyptus, spruce, lily and in foods such as mulberries, peanuts, resveratrol's most abundant natural sources are vitis vinifera, labrusca, and muscadine grapes, which are used to make wines. It occurs in the vines, roots, seeds and stalks, but its highest concentration is in the grape skins, which contain about 50-100 mcg/ per gram.

6. "Coffee, The Potent Brew"

Coffee, by some studies, may be one of our lead sources of fighting disease. It contains fighting antioxidants and in one study by the University of Scranton, suggests that the average adult gets 4 times as many antioxidants from coffee as from tea and 15 times more than bananas, beans and corn. One of the best antioxidant coffees, 'java', helps reduce cell damage, aging, reduce risk of cancer and heart disease.

7. Aspartame Low Calorie Sweetener (Equal), Is It Safe?

Most studies argue that aspartame is indeed safe as a low calorie sweetener. It is composed of two amino acids, aspartic acid and phenylalanine, as a mild ester. Amino acids are the building blocks of protein. Aspartic acid and phenylalanine are also found naturally in protein containing foods such as meats, grains, and dairy products. Methyl esters are also found naturally in many foods such as fruits, vegetables, and their juices. A large scale 'NIH-AARP' Diet and Health Study" found that those who drink beverages with aspartame have no greater risk of brain cancer, lymphoma,, or leukemia than those who do not.

8. Do You Have What It Takes To Live Beyond 100 years? What Does It Take?

1-Runs in the family!

Centenarians tend to have parents and grandparents who live or who have lived a very long time.

2-Diseases later in life!

Centenarians, who get life-threatening diseases 20 or 30 years later in life than the rest of the population, could possess a slower rate of aging process.

3-Don't worry!

Psychologically, centenarians tend to be more relaxed, optimistic, even-tempered and not the type-a personality.

4-Is big better?-Lipoproteins!

Big is better. The size of centenarian lipoproteins-the molecules that carry cholesterol within the blood, are much larger than the average. In the war against heart disease, large lipoproteins are thought to be better protectors.

5-Good cholesterol (HDL)!

The offspring of centenarians frequently have extremely high levels of 'good cholesterol' or HDL. It is likely than when younger, centenarians also had high HDL levels which may have protected them from heart disease.

6-Are you lucky or more Blessed?

Let's face it, some folks are just lucky or blessed. It turns out that many centenarians do not lead a healthy lifestyle. About 30 percent were overweight and some were even smokers.

9. In Order To Lose Weight, How Many Calories Are Burned With Exercise?

Diet plans, especially 'fads' usually don't last. A solid exercise plan can really help not only with better weight control, but it may actually 'reverse' or at least slow down the aging process.

It is preferred that you choose one of the 30-60-90 minute rule plans. Work out daily at least 5 days per week. It's a smart plan and it works.

Running indoors or using a treadmill or elliptical running, all of these, are some of the best calorie burners, but watch the knees. Don't forget about walking. It is also a very good way to exercise. Here is a exercise list of **"Calories To Burn"**.

Calories To Burn Per Hour, by Body Weight:

Cal/120 pounds versus cal/170 pounds: here we have a 120 pound person and a 170 pound person:

1. Running (10 mph)-880 cal/1,230 cal
2. Indoor cycling-hard-572 cal/810 cal
3. Skiing, cross country-440 cal/615 cal
4. Rowing, stationary-385 cal/540 cal

5. Skating, roller-385 cal/540 cal
6. Skiing, downhill-385 cal/540 cal
7. Soccer-385 cal/540 cal
8. Tennis-385 cal/540 cal
9. Aerobic dance-330 cal/460 cal
10. Basketball-330 cal/460 cal
11. Hiking-330 cal/460 cal
12. Swimming, leisure-330 cal/460 cal
13. Golf (walking)-250 cal/345 cal
14. Bicycling (under 10 mph)-220 cal/310 cal
15. Walking, brisk-220 cal/310 cal
16. Weight training, light-165 cal/230 cal
17. Sitting (watching TV)-55 cal/75 cal

10. "Overdosed America" (by Dr. John Abramson, Comments):

"Truth is, lifestyle is more important than cholesterol levels. About 70% of our health has to do with how we live our lives. Doctors are not keeping up with this. Only America and New Zealand allow direct to consumer advertising." The powerful pharmaceutical companies blast the television, magazines, newspapers, and any media available with high powered ads enticing the public to call their doctor and say they want to try this medicine, they "saw on television". The real sad result is that most doctors, 50-80%, give in and write or call in a prescription as the customer wanted.

11. "Your Body's Abundant Bacteria" –You're Not Going To Believe This!

Ever wonder why the space aliens (in theory) rather quickly perished, after they breathed earth's air, like in the movies, "War of the Worlds"? Ever wonder why, after Columbus introduced the new world to the old, with thousands of "New Americans" and their wheat, horses, pigs, and their sugarcane, rice and slaves, that between 1492 and 1650, the entire indigenous population of North and South America perished by 90%, due to smallpox, measles, and other old world diseases?

Ever wonder why nearly 20 million people died with the plague in the early 1900's (1918-1920)?

Research into bacteria and how much we as humans actually carry at any one time may be controversial, but it is generally agreed that we carry up to "millions" or more. Here is a review of where we keep these bacteria and comments about them. In one report, by 'Discover' in November, 2005, it was suggested that the human body may contain 100 trillion bacteria! And they are not just partners! They aid in digesting your food, help make vitamins, protect you from dangerous pathogens and may even play a role in regulating your appetite and weight.

1-Eyes:

The tears contain natural antibiotics that kill most organisms. But they are also a home to several harmless strains of stapyloccous which help prevent the more virulent strains from causing many eye infections.

2-Ears:

Even though certain waxy secretions contain antibacterial components there may exist more than 200 bacterial species in the outer ear.

3-Nose:

It is estimated that 20% of us carry a more virulent strain of staphyloccus aureus, which is normally not a problem unless a cut lets the bacteria in the blood stream which then can become very serious and in some cases, fatal. The nose harbors many less harmful bacteria which buffer the potential pathogens, especially streptococcus pneumonia.

4-Mouth:

Research suggests, that the mouth may contain up to 500 different microbial species. They harbor in your teeth, plaque, and can easily cause bad breath and cavities.

5-Skin:

Human skin is generally low in moisture, and its low ph and high salinity make it inhospitable for all except for a few bacteria.

6-Armpits:

Most of the trillions (twelve trillion) or so skin bacteria prefer the moist environments of the armpits, groin, where urea, protein, salts and lactic acid leak out of sweat glands and also gather in hair follicles.

7-Stomach:

In the past, it was thought that the stomach was too acidic to host any life, but we know today, that the bacterium heliobacter pylori does exist and may cause ulcers in some folks.

8-Small Intestine:

Fortunately, bile and antimicrobial mucus help keep the small intestine sparsely populated. However, certain strains of streptococci, bifidobacteria, clostridia may remain. In a 2002 study, it was discovered that bacteroides thetaiotamicron sends signals needed for the blood vessels of the bowels to develop properly after birth.

9-Colon:

The colon may contain up to 2 pounds of bacteria! (this amount is controversial). It is said, that the bacteria in the colon make up to 1/3 of feces weight. The different types of bacteria Help metabolize bile acids, break down indigestible parts of our food and produce Vitamin K and B-12.

10-Urinary tract:

The urethra is normally quite sterile, except for the ½ inch near the exit. Urinary tract infections occur when certain strains of the colon-dwelling escherichia coli bacteria and colonize at the opening and upward.

11-Reproductive tract:

Several species of lactobacillus help keep the vagina slight acidic ph. If the bacteria are killed, the ph goes up and promotes the overgrowth of candida fungas.

12-Feet:

Many moisture loving bacteria thrive between the toes.

13-Sterile areas: (no bacteria)

The following areas are normally sterile: liver, gall bladder, brain, thymus, blood, and lower lungs.

12. "Men Need To Overcome Workout Barriers"-by Jorge Cruise. Comments:

1-Men generally die about 6 years younger than women

2-Men have higher death rates from all but one of 15 leading causes of death

3-Many men make health and fitness a low priority

4-Will Courtenay, director of Men's Health in Berkeley, California, says: "we can talk to men about exercise and health till we are blue in the face, but it won't matter if attitudes don't change"

5-Three things you can do to get started (improve your health and fitness):

First, get a checkup (and get one every year). Secondly, re-examine your fitness plan. Is it working or do you have one? And thirdly, (his favorite) set up a workout plan, 30 minutes a day of challenging cardio, 5 days a week and 30 minutes a day with 'resistance' training, 3 days a week. And spend one day committed to spending time with your wife and children, with some type of physical activity included.

13. Ginger, Red Chilli Peppers May Show Promise Against Cancer.

"We found that ginger induced cell death at a similar or better rate than platinum-based chemotherapy drugs used to treat ovarian cancer"-by Dr. Jennifer Rhode

1-Studies are showing, that ginger and the hot element in red chili peppers induce tumor cells to die

2-Capsaicin, the hot ingredient in pepper, causes pancreatic cancer cells to die through the body's normal process for clearing defective cells

3-Tumors treated with capsaicin were half the size of tumors (found in mice) that were treated with saline solution.

4-Ginger caused cell death in all the ovarian-cancer cells in lines tested. In addition, the spice caused cancer cells to be destroyed both through the normal cell-death process and through another mechanism that involves the cells digesting themselves from the inside out

5-Ginger is known to be helpful in controlling inflammation and inflammation contributes to the development of ovarian cancer cells. By stopping the inflammation, ginger also stops the cancer cells from growing.

6-In a study by the national cancer institute, researchers said that while soy intake may reduce the risk of breast cancer, the evidence may be too weak to recommend for widespread use.

14. Licorice, Glycyrrhic acid, a compound in licorice, may have anti-sarcoma cancer and other amazing properties:

1-One of the world's oldest known medicines (licorice root)

2-Historically it has been used to treat colds, asthma and used for healing wounds

3-Herbalists in China and India add licorice to their compounds to remedy sore throats

4-Recently, scientists worldwide are testing Glycyrrhic acid and some have found that it kills cancer cells that cause Kaposi's sarcoma.

5-It also inhibits growth of the Sars (severe acute respiratory syndrome) virus and has been successful against Japanese encephalitis, chronic hepatitis and HIV.

15. Is Your "Tap Water" That Pure?-study by Chloe Chitwood, Comments:

1-Tap water in more than 40 states is contaminated

2-The most widely used disinfectant is chlorine, which when broken down, forms trithalomethanes, which are known carcinogens (cancer causing agents) and contribute to colon stomach and other cancers

3-Other chemicals are added to water to keep solids in suspension and some of these are carcinogens. Pharmaceuticals, hormones, oral contraceptives and even Prozac are found in tap drinking water

4-Most commercial ice is contaminated and may contain bacteria and debris

5-Harris poll in 2005 stated that water pollution was the number one concern facing the country. Even more than global warming and ozone depletion

6-More modern use of ultraviolet light as a disinfectant may be a much better way to achieve better drinking water. In some Midwestern and Eastern states, ultraviolet light is used to purify water. Millions of gallons of water can be purified at one time. Ultraviolet light destroys the DNA of bacteria and keeps them from replicating. The "UV" light also destroys parasites. The best thing about UV light is, after the water has passed through the unit, the water has been disinfected, and the quality is pure.

7-Ozone water treatment is another form of purification, which has the same germicidal effect as UV, but it may also cause corrosion of metal parts

8-About 60% of water pollution results from urban sprawl and industrial chemicals

9-Osmotic filters filter out particles and traps them, but they must be changed frequently. There are several lesser filters that trap only larger particles. Filters do not destroy bacteria.

10-The purer process for pure water is water distillation. Water is boiled, then distilled and condensed in a container. This process destroys more than 95% of pollutants, including bacteria

11-Water is very important to health. Pure water helps keep heavy metals, such as lead, from remaining in our lower extremities. Removing solids from water, aids in preventing atherosclerosis.

12-More and more diseases, even reproductive toxicity, are found to be attributable to contaminated water. Examples of potential diseases are autism, birth defects, and brain cancer.

Drink Purified Water!

16. Dangers of Trans-Fatty Acids: (by Kathleen McGowan, comments)

1-A study at Wake Forrest, in North Carolina revealed that even small amounts of trans fats lead to a serious condition of weight gain, atherosclerosis and insulin resistance (in monkeys)

2-Trans fats are the partially hydrogenated vegetable oils in cooking containers in most fast food chains. They use this 'oil' preparation because they are more shelf-life stable and are resistant to high heat.

3-In recent years, evidence has shown that these trans-fats contribute to heart disease, rather quickly, and high cholesterol, and type 2 diabetes

4-Comments from the New England Journal of Medicine, Walter Willett at the Harvard School of Public Health, exclaimed that "trans-fats are probably a bigger public health problem than either food contamination or pesticides…trans fats are clearly toxic to humans and have no place in human diets".

17. Is Catching Some Rays, A Good Idea?

There has been and there still is, a warning, stay out of the sun, without protection, because of the greater risk of skin cancer. But according to Michael Holic, MD and PHD, Boston University Medical Center, sunlight is our primary source of Vitamin D. Spending a small amount of time in direct sunlight, without a sunscreen, can help ward off serious illnesses, including diabetes, heart disease, multiple sclerosis, rheumatoid arthritis, osteoporosis, and even some cancers. When you wear a sunscreen, it reduces the production of Vitamin D in the skin. The Vitamin D supplements may not contain enough health-protecting D-3 nutrient that comes from sunshine.

By sunning your unprotected face, arms and hands for a **few minutes,** you can produce as much Vitamin D as is in ten glasses of milk. The darker your skin is, the longer it may take.

With fair skin, it is recommended, to spend 5-10 minutes in the sun, two or three times per week. If your skin is dark, spend 15-30 minutes.

However, more is not better. If you are going to sunbathe for longer periods than suggested above, then apply a sunscreen. After you sunbathe, apply more sunscreen and reapply every 2 hours for as long as you are outdoors.

18. Fish Meals, Weekly, Boosts Brain Health

It is recommended to eat fish at least once a week, for several reasons, but one is that it is good for the brain, and helps slow age-related decline by the equivalent of three to four years!

There is growing evidence that a fish-rich diet helps keep the mind sharp.

Other previous studies, found that people who ate fish, lowered their risk of alzheimer's disease and stroke.

19. Eat A Breakfast Every Day!

1-People who skip breakfast are 4 and ½ times more likely to be overweight than those who don't.

2-Oatmeal versus Granola versus Farina (cream of wheat) :

Granola is really a snack food and is not considered a healthy breakfast. Cream of wheat is short on calories, not including the sugars you might add. But oatmeal is packed with nutritional pluses, including protein, iron, magnesium, zinc, manganese, thiamin and fiber. It may also help lower cholesterol levels, and reduce the risk of heart disease. Just be careful what you add. Brown sugar, butter, honey and whole milk can make a healthy meal, not healthy.

3-Sausage versus Bacon versus Ham:

Ham is the winner because of its low calories and low saturated fat (but watch the salt). Bacon is not a great choice. At least with sausage, you probably won't eat too many. Try turkey bacon.

4-Waffles versus Pancakes versus French Toast:

Waffles and pancakes are not too bad, as long as you are careful what you add. French toast is considered less healthy, because of the extra calories. Suggest using whole-wheat flour for your pancakes and whole wheat bread for your French toast. Also, you can make your French toast with egg whites. Also, adding fresh fruit can make your meal more nutritious.

5-Muffins versus Scones versus Croissants:

A plain croissant may be your best choice. Croissants are usually packed with butter, and scones and muffins are typically large, individually baked pieces of cake. May be better to split a muffin with another person

20. The Obvious Key To Living Longer Is To Eat Less!

Eating less, slows down the metabolism and that alone prolongs life. Obesity and diabetes shorten life span. When people eat too much all too often, the body is stressed by insulin overproduction. The rising insulin levels cause obesity and increase the risk of diabetes, heart disease, and other psychological changes that age the organs and reduce life span.

21. Practical Strategies For Delaying or Preventing The Onset of Alzheimer's Disease:

1-Increase active brain functions, by learning new activities, reading, socializing and games

2-Take or eat lots of antioxidants such as Vitamin C, Vitamin E, grape seed, blueberries, strawberries, drink green tea (and chew and eat some of the leaves), spinach, with lots of fruits and vegetables

3-Take multivitamins especially with all the B vitamins, folic acid, and minerals

4-Daily exercise 30, 60 or 90 minutes per day and good sleep hygiene

5-Caloric restriction (1,600-1,700 per day), weight reduction and fewer refined carbohydrates and less saturated fats and no trans fats

6-Lower blood pressure

7-Lower cholesterol, LDL and raise HDL

8-Treat and or avoid depression, anxiety, and stress

9-Increase Omega-3 polyunsaturated fatty acids

10-Limit alcohol intake to 2 drinks per day

11-Lower weight and prevent periodontal disease

22. Live Longer!

A landmark study of more than 17,000 middle-aged Harvard graduates found that those who regularly exercise, vigorously, reduced their risk of dying prematurely by at least 25%. This was thought to be due to those that exercise, have a lower risk of having a heart attack or stroke. It was also found, that the more vigorously you exercise, the longer you will live! "The reason why we don't live longer isn't because of the way we are made, its because we don't take care of ourselves" (says Kenneth Cooper, MD, Executive Director of the Cooper Institute of Aerobic Research in Dallas). He goes on to say, "Our bodies should last us 120 years".

23. Extra Benefits from Exercise!

1-You already know exercise is good for you and that regular physical activity can reduce risk of developing heart disease, diabetes, alzheimer's disease and some forms of cancer.

2-Did you know that exercise can actually decrease pain in people with arthritis?

3-Women who exercise vigorously experience far fewer hot flashes that those who don't.

4-"If you could put exercise in a pill, you'd be able to treat so many chronic conditions and diseases", says Roger Fielding, PHD, Director of Nutrition and Exercise Physiology Lab at Tuft University.

5-Aerobic exercise (strenuous exercises that produce a marked temporary increase in respiration and heart rate) stimulates the cardiovascular system, boosting blood flow to the heart and the rest of the body. Researchers believe many of the health benefits attributed to aerobic exercise stem from this increased blood flow.

24. A Banana A Day, Helps Keep The Doctor Away!

1-A banana contains 3 natural sugars-sucrose, fructose and glucose and also contains some fiber.

2-A banana can give an instant boost of energy and in fact, 2 bananas a day can provide enough energy for a strenuous 90 minute workout!

3-Bananas are the #one fruit with world athletes

4-Bananas help overcome or prevent a substantial number of illnesses and conditions, making it a must in our daily diet

5-People suffering from depression, felt better after eating a banana, this is because of it contains tryptophan, a type of protein that the body converts into serotonin, known to make you relax, improve your mood and generally make you feel happier

6-Bananas can stimulate the production of hemoglobin in the blood and therefore helps in cases of anemia

7-Help lower blood pressure. This unique tropical fruit is extremely high in potassium, yet low in salt which makes it a perfect way to help maintain better blood pressure

8-Assists in improving brain power and make the pupils more alert

9-Bananas are high in fiber and help restore normal bowel action and help relieve constipation

10-Bananas have a natural soothing antacid relief and help relieve heartburn

11-Snacking between meals with bananas helps keep blood sugar levels up and avoid morning sickness

12-Before using an insect bite cream, rub the affected area with the inside of a banana skin and it reduces the swelling and irritation

13-Bananas are high in "B" vitamins that can help calm the nervous system

14-Bananas can be used as a dietary food against intestinal disorders because of its soft texture and smoothness. It also neutralizes over acidity and reduces irritation by coating the stomach. Also helps reduce the effects of ulcers

15-Many other cultures see bananas as a 'cooling fruit' that can lower both the physical and emotional temperature of expectant mothers. In Thailand, pregnant women eat bananas to ensure their baby is born with a cool temperature

16-Bananas help seasonal affective disorder ('sad) sufferers because they contain a natural mood enhancer, tryptophan

17-People who smoke, may find bananas help them give up smoking. The B-6, B-12, potassium and magnesium help the body recover from the effects of nicotine withdrawal

18-Potassium, high in content in bananas, it a vital mineral, which helps normalize the heartbeat, sends oxygen to the brain and regulates your body's water balance

19-Strokes-according to the New England Journal of Medicine, eating bananas as part of a regular diet can cut the risk of death by strokes as much as 40%

20-So, a banana really is a natural remedy for many ills. When compared to an apple, it has 4 times the protein, twice the carbohydrates, 3 times the phosphorous, 5 times the Vitamin A and iron, and twice the amount of vitamins and minerals and is also rich in potassium. It is also one of the best food values anywhere.

25. Some of The Best Healthy Foods Are:

Some of the best nutritional and healing foods that are natural and have no side effects are (says Gabrielle De Groat Redford): **whole grains, cherries, yogurt, salmon, cabbage, walnuts, blueberries, beans and tomatoes.**

1-Whole grains:

Whole grains have a bunch of phytonutrients (parts of plants that have health benefits) that are just as nutritious as fruits and vegetables (says Susan Moores, a Minneapolis Nutritionist and spokesperson for the American Dietetic Association). According the University of Minnesota, eating 3 daily servings of whole grains can reduce the risk of heart disease by 25-36 %, stroke by 37% and type-2 diabetes by 21 to 27 %. Whole grains include oats, whole wheat, brown rice, bulgur (a Middle Eastern, Indian, and Mediterranean wheat species, whole grain and hi-fiber) and bran.

2-Cherries:

Scientists, studying the link between diet and disease often look for a "marker" in the blood called "C-reactive protein" or "CRP". The CRP is produced in the body in response to acute inflammation, like that which occurs with arthritis sufferers. In a study done by the 'Western Human Nutrition Research Center in Davis, California", volunteers were asked to eat a bowl of cherries (45 fresh) and then their CRP was measured and it was found that the 'CRP' levels decreased. In The Encyclopedia of Healing Foods, Simon and Schuster, 2005, one of the old-time therapies for gout (a painful type of arthritis) was black cherries. Of course, 45 cherries at one meal is too many, but adding antioxidant-rich cherries to your diet a couple of times a week can be helpful.

3-Yogurt:

"Probiotics" are the friendly bacteria that when eaten, help fight illness or disease. Yogurt is the most popular food containing 'probiotics'. Two recent studies found that eating yogurt improves a person's ability to fight off pneumonia.

4-Salmon:

Salmon is loaded with heart-healthy omega-3 fatty acids. Adding salmon to your diet can help lower cholesterol, lower blood pressure and help prevent heart disease. Recently, University of California at San Diego, have reported that higher intake of omega-3's appear to preserve bone density, helping keep your bones stronger and protecting against falls and fractures. Jennifer Sacheck, PHD., Assistant Professor of Nutrition Science and Policy at Tufts University, says, " these fish, salmon, sardines, tuna and mackerel, are high in omega-3's and people who consume them have a lower risk of heart attack, hypertension and stroke".

5-Cabbage:

Cabbage may help protect against breast cancer. Other studies have found that cabbage may also protect against lung, stomach, and colon cancers.

6-Walnuts:

Walnuts also contain healthy amounts of omega-3's, which also help reduce the risk of heart disease and hypertension. In one study, Japanese men and women who ate ¼ - 1/3 cup of walnuts per day, lowered their bad "LDL" cholesterol levels by 10%. Walnuts (and almonds, and pistachios) are high in arginine, an amino acid that increases blood flow to the heart.

7-Blueberries:

Recent studies show that eating plenty of blueberries may help lessen brain damage from strokes and may reduce the effects of alzheimer's disease or dementia. Blueberries help keep the mind sharp. In one research study at USDA Human Nutrition Research Center on Aging at Tufts University, 40 fruits and vegetables were tested for their disease-fighting antioxidant activity and blueberries not only came out on top, but were just as powerful as two to three servings of other fruits and vegetables.

8-Beans:

There have been several studies suggesting that beans are not only a great source of protein and antioxidants, but because of their higher fiber, they help reduce the risk of colon cancer. In a study published by the Journal of American Medical Association, a healthy diet rich in lean protein, about half from plant sources such as beans, was found to lower blood pressure, lower 'bad' LDL cholesterol, and to cut the risk of heart disease by 21%.

9-Tomatoes:

It has been known for many years that tomatoes are a healthy food source. Regular eating tomato-based foods can reduce a man's risk of prostate cancer by up to 35 %. More recently, studies have shown that men who already have prostate cancer may also benefit as well.

26. Walking The Dog and Drop 14 Pounds In A Year!

Researchers at the University of Missouri-Columbia found that sedentary folks who took up the habit of walking the dog, not only lost weight, they also improved their flexibility and balance and felt better about themselves. "Adding a dog to your daily walk, can even spur die-hard couch potatoes to change their ways, says Rebecca Johnson, PHD., Professor of Gerontological Nursing".

27. Long Term Stress Leads To Premature Aging of Various Cells!

Short term stress can actually be a good thing, says Bruce McEwen, PHD., head of Neuroendocrinology Laboratories at Rockefeller University. "Stress is a positive experience if there is a feeling of control and satisfaction. You need challenges".

Long term stress, the kind you can't control or resolve, can have far-reaching harmful consequences. Recent research at the University of California, San Francisco, has shown that chronic stress appears to shorten 'telomeres', the caps at the end of our chromosomes. This leads to premature aging of our cells.

Long term stress speeds up atherosclerosis (clogging of the arteries), and too much cortisol damages brain cells. "There is evidence that elevated levels of stress hormones cause the hippocampus, which is the crucial moderator of memory, to atrophy, says Marilyn Albert, PHD., a Neurology Professor at Johns Hopkins University."

28. Height (Feet and Inches) Weight (Pounds) Chart:

Females	Females	Females	Females	Males	Males	Males	Males
Height	Low	Target	High	Height	Low	Target	High
4'10"	100	115	131	5'1"	123	134	145
4'11"	101	117	134	5'2"	125	137	148
5'0"	103	120	137	5'3"	127	139	151
5'1"	105	122	140	5'4"	129	142	155
5'2"	108	125	144	5'5"	131	145	159
5'3"	111	128	148	5'6"	133	148	163
5'4"	114	133	152	5'7"	135	151	167
5'5"	117	136	156	5'8"	137	154	171
5'6"	120	140	160	5'9"	139	157	175
5'7"	123	143	164	5'10"	141	160	179
5'8"	126	146	167	5'11"	144	164	183
5'9"	129	150	170	6'0"	147	167	187
5'10"	132	153	173	6'1"	150	171	192
5'11"	135	156	176	6'2"	153	175	197
6'0"	138	159	179	6'3"	157	179	202

Comments Regarding These Special Reports and Reviews:

This series of reports and reviews are offered for your review. Throughout the book, we have emphasized the importance of exercise, importance of antioxidants, and vitamins, minerals, weight control, diet control, watching and evaluating the seven food factors-calories, cholesterol, fat, carbohydrates, fiber, protein and salt. More and more research supports the consumption of fruits and vegetables, fish, nuts and whole grain products to prolong and enhance longevity as well as a healthy life. Your choice of Lifestyle is what it is all about. Choose wisely and you will live a lot longer.

Special thanks to my wonderful wife, Therese Legare, and my very special son, Sean. Their patience and support will always be appreciated and loved.

JOHN WILLIAM KELLY

.